Rodrigo Giuberti

Bond Strength of Resin Cement to Titanium and Zir Surfaces

Rodrigo Giuberti

Bond Strength of Resin Cement to Titanium and Zir Surfaces

Aluminum Oxide Blasting for Surface Treatment of Titanium and Zinc Oxide

ScienciaScripts

Imprint

Cover image: www.ingimage.com

This book is a translation from the original published under ISBN 978-613-9-62804-9.

Publisher:
Sciencia Scripts
is a trademark of
Dodo Books Indian Ocean Ltd. and OmniScriptum S.R.L publishing group

120 High Road, East Finchley, London, N2 9ED, United Kingdom
Str. Armeneasca 28/1, office 1, Chisinau MD-2012, Republic of Moldova, Europe
Printed at: see last page
ISBN: 978-620-7-75122-8

SUMMARY

ACKNOWLEDGMENTS

I thank God for the opportunity to take this course and for helping me in my quest for knowledge.

To my parents Gilson Giuberti (in memoriam) and Zélia Ferreira Giuberti for their support and encouragement throughout my life.

To my children Breno and Hanna, for always being part of my story.

To my brothers Gilson, Luiz Guilherme and Moema for the support I always receive and for believing in me.

The Sao Leopoldo Mandic School, which welcomed me for my master's degree, enabling me to grow and be recognized in my professional career.

To Prof. Dr. Geraldo Alberto, for his contribution to my work and tips on my professional career.

To the teachers of this team coordinated by Prof. Dr. Sérgio Candido Dias for the dynamics of the course and the quality of the lectures.

To Prof.[a] . Dr. Cecilia Turssi for having collaborated in this work and for her formidable teaching.

To Laboratório Padilha (Vitória/ES) for their participation in the milling of the Zirconium Oxide samples.

Singular Dalton (Natal/RN) for supplying the grade V titanium samples.

SUMMARY

Surface treatment methods have been developed and tested for effective bonding between the cementing agent and the surface of the Zirconium Oxide ceramic, but there is no consensus on a methodology. The aim of this study was to evaluate the shear bond strength of two resin cements to the surface of titanium and zirconium oxide ceramics, taking into account the treatment and non-treatment of their respective surfaces. Zirconium oxide ceramic stabilized with itrium oxide and grade V titanium alloy was used. The cementation systems used were RelyX U200 (Self-Adhesive Resin Cement) and Multilink Sistem Pack (Self-Curing Resin Cement). A total of 80 samples (N = 80) were used to form the zirconia (N = 40) and titanium (N = 40) groups. The groups were subdivided into eight subgroups (n = 10) as follows: G 1 = Zr treated U200; G 2 = Zr not treated U200; G 3= Zr treated Multilink; G 4 = Zr not treated Multilink; G 5= Ti treated U200; G 6= Ti not treated U200; G 7 = Ti treated Multilink; G 8 = Ti not treated Multilink. The samples were fabricated, prepared with aluminum oxide blasting, metal/zirconia primer applied and cemented. They were subjected to 1000 thermal cycles of artificial ageing and a shear bond strength test. The bond strength values were subjected to three-way analysis of variance and the failure modes observed in the samples were analyzed descriptively. The self-adhesive cement RelyX U200 achieved good results only on the titanium samples where it was surface treated, and was not effective on zirconium regardless of the surface treatment. The surface treatment with aluminum oxide blasting associated with Metal/Zirconia Primer and Multilink cement was sufficient to increase the bond strength values of cementation on the Titanium surface, while it was not effective on the Zirconia surface.

Keywords: Surface treatment. Bond strength. Resin cement.

DISSEMINATION AND TRANSFER OF KNOWLEDGE

The aim of this study was to evaluate the strength of two adhesive glues on a Titanium metal and a Zirconium Oxide ceramic surface. For this purpose, forty square pieces of Zirconium Oxide and forty round pieces of Titanium were made, three millimeters thick and approximately five square millimeters in area. All these pieces underwent surface treatment such as sanding with a polishing machine, blasting with aluminum oxide particles and air, blasting with air and water, cleaning in an ultrasonic tank with distilled water and bonding with the two cements selected for this study. After all the bonding was done, the pieces were subjected to an artificial ageing process and mechanical testing by specific machines. The results obtained after the mechanical test were analyzed and concluded.

1 INTRODUCTION

Zirconium oxide ceramics have been widely used in dentistry to make metal-free fixed partial dentures, due to their good and satisfactory optical properties, biocompatibility, low thermal conductivity, chemical stability, as well as their high resistance to fracture and mechanical performance when compared to other types of dental ceramics. Its clinical applications include ceramic cores, indirect inlay and onlay restorations, copings, orthodontic brackets, dental implants and as an infrastructure for fixed crowns and bridges. The disadvantage of this material is that it degrades due to ageing at low temperatures and degradation in aqueous environments such as water vapor, humidity and the presence of fluids (Kern, Thompson, 1994; Manicone et al., 2007; Aboushelib et al, 2009; Wolfart et al., 2009; Mirmohammadi et al., 2010; Qeblawi et al., 2010; Attia, Kern, 2010; Miyazaki et al., 2013; Belo et al., 2013; Fragoso et al., 2015; Satake et al., 2015; El-Ghany et al., 2016; Tzanakakis et al., 2016).

With the evolution of fabrication systems and materials, the clinical, mechanical and aesthetic success of metal-free all-ceramic pieces is still heavily dependent on the bonding process (Thompson et al., 2011; Belo et al., 2013; Miyazaki et al., 2013; Inokoshi et al., 2014; Papia et al., 2014; El-Ghany & Sherief, 2016; Hallmann et al., 2016; Tzanakakis et al., 2016). The composition and microstructure of ceramics, associated with the physical and chemical properties of cementing agents, significantly influence the bonding mechanism and durability of ceramic restorations (Piconi, Maccauro, 1999; Ozcan, Vallittu 2003; Yun et al., 2010; Mosele, Borba, 2014; Della Bona et al., 2015; Pozzobon et al., 2017). The adhesion of resin cements to zirconia is more difficult when compared to feldspathic ceramics, as they have a higher vitreous phase content. For feldspathic ceramics, the use of hydrofluoric acid and the application of a silane agent have traditionally proved to be more effective, with high strength and longevity values. However, for zirconium, this method does not guarantee satisfactory adhesion due to its high crystalline phase content and lack of glass (Thompson et al., 2011; Lung et al., 2015; Hallmann et al., 2016; Tzanakakis et al., 2016).

Obtaining adhesion of resin cements to the inner surface of zirconia requires specific preparation in order to promote a retentive surface and reliable chemical bonding (Kern, Thompson, 1994; Ozcan, Vallittu, 2003; Tsuchimoto et al, 2006; Wolfart et al., 2007; Mosele, Borba, 2014; Satake et al., 2015; Tzanakakis et al., 2016; Satake et al., 2015; Pozzobon et al., 2017). To promote adhesion of the substrate to the zirconium surface, we have mechanical treatment, chemical treatment, the use of lasers, coating techniques with silica particles, the use of coupling agents and initiating agents present in cements. Surface treatment consists of the formation of mechanical retention associated with the application of a coupling agent in order to bond the resin cement to the zirconium surface (Aboushelib et al., 2009; Mirmohammadi et al., 2010; Satake et al., 2015; Ozcan, Bernasconi, 2015; Tzanakakis et al., 2016; Pozzobon et al., 2017).

Since there are concerns about the possible damage created by physical treatment methods to promote retention, some manufacturers have started to produce initiating agents and resin cements based on organophosphates, such as carboxylic acid monomers and phosphate esters, specific for zirconium, which could eliminate more aggressive conditioning methods. However, the hydrolytic degradation of silanes, initiating agents and acidic monomers is still problematic, as the hydrolysis of silanes and initiators in water reduces their performance, limiting their useful life (Ozcan, Bernasconi, 2015). (Thompson et al., 2011; Della Bona et al., 2015; El-Ghany & Sherief, 2016; Hallmann et al., 2016; Tzanakakis et al., 2016).

Studies have shown that the adhesion capacity of dental cements to the internal surface of zirconium oxide ceramics has been unsatisfactory. Therefore, there must be a correct association between the type of mechanical surface treatment and the type of resin system, as many factors can influence the results of studies, such as the aging methodology, types of tests used in the experiment, surface topography and possible damage to the zirconium surface as a result of mechanical treatment (Mosele, Borba, 2014; Satake et al., 2015; Hallmann et al., 2016). Due to the wide variety of surface treatment methods and types of bonding agents, it is necessary to identify evidence that can support the use of a reliable technique for bonding. To date, there is no consensus on the best surface treatment method to achieve a good and durable bond between resin cement and zirconium oxide ceramic (Mosele, Borba, 2014; Satake et al., 2015; Hallmann et al., 2016; Pozzobon et al., 2017).

The aim of this study was to evaluate the shear bond strength of two different resin cement systems, Multilink self-curing cement (IVOCLAIR Vivadent) and U200 self-adhesive cement (3M ESPE), to grade V titanium and a ceramic made of zirconium oxide stabilized with itrium oxide, both treated and untreated.

2 LITERATURE REVIEW

Kern & Thompson (1994) evaluated the effects of blasting and coating techniques on volume loss, surface morphology and compositional changes in pure titanium. Coating the titanium surface with silica improves the chemical-mechanical bond, as blasting is recommended as a pre-treatment. Volume loss was similar to values reported for titanium-based alloys and does not appear to be critical for the clinical fit of restorations. After tribochemical silica coating, a small amount of silica particles remained loose on the surface and ultrasonic cleaning removed all loose silica and aluminum particles from the surface. The low content of loose alumina or silica suggests that most of the alumina and silica are fixed to the titanium surface. The silica content following the coating treatment increased by only 1.4% by weight of the sandblasted sample. The silica layer employed by these coating methods differs widely in both morphology and thickness. These results provide a basis for explaining adhesive failure modes in bond strength tests and for developing methods for adhesive cementation. Clinically, ultrasonic cleaning of titanium and chemical tribo coating of silica should improve resin bonding and remove loose particles, without relevant changes in composition.

Taira et al. (1998) carried out a study to investigate the influence of titanium surface oxidation on the strength and durability of the bond with the cementing agent. A cementing agent and a methacrylate-phosphate (MDP) initiator were used in this study. Two groups of Ti samples were fabricated by machining and casting in which they underwent surface treatment forming three subgroups: 1) Cast; 2) Polished; 3) Aluminum oxide blast after polishing. After preparing the discs, they were ultrasonically cleaned in distilled water for 10 minutes and air-dried. These samples were placed in an electric oven (Accu-therm II 500[a] , Japan) for 10 minutes at temperatures of 400, 500, 600, 700 and 800°C and then allowed to cool to room temperature. All this was done to induce an individual oxidation characteristic on the surface and these samples were divided into distinct groups. A piece of adhesive tape with a 5 mm diameter hole was positioned on the surface of each sample to outline the bonding area and to define the reliable shape of the adhesive area. The cementing agent was applied to the titanium surface and an acrylic rod (6 mm in diameter and 5 mm thick) was affixed. After 30 minutes of preparation, the samples were immersed in water at 37°C for twenty-four hours, considering this stage as pre-thermocycling. Parts of the samples were thermocycled alternating between 4 and 60°C for a period of 5,000 cycles. The samples were subjected to a shear strength test and the results were analyzed by analysis of variance (ANOVA) and surface flaws were assessed using an optical microscope (SMZ-10 NIKOIU, Japan). The thin layer of oxide produced by the atmosphere on this metal alloy allows monomer derived from carboxylic or phosphoric acids to produce strong adhesive bonds, but too much can interfere with the durability of the bond. The surface treatment, using an aluminium oxide jet, had an adequate durability and resistance, and an excess of the oxide layer on the surface reduces the durability of the cementation, as the work concludes.

McCracken (1999) reviewed the literature describing the properties of commercially pure titanium and titanium alloys, with a view to their impact on the choice of treatment. Titanium has biocompatibility, corrosion resistance, good ductility, high tensile strength and reasonable machinability. Like steel, it has two phases in its atomic structure: hexagonal (stable up to 882°C) and cubic phase above 882°C. The stability of these phases is due to the addition of certain elements such as manganese, chromium, iron and vanadium. Titanium is presented as commercially pure titanium [Ti-CP], in its pure form, and in various grades (titanium alloy), where its composition is altered, changing the physical properties according to the purposes available in these alloys. For use in dental implants, studies have shown with clinical evidence that all the materials available for dental implants exhibit excellent biocompatibility, good tissue response and predictability. The conclusion is that no titanium-based material has proven to be more biocompatible than any other group and that in the absence of comparative studies, factors such as implant design, size and material strength should determine implant selection for a given patient. Independent studies should be carried out to evaluate these effects.

Piconi & Maccauro (1999) published a literature review in which they reported on the use of zirconium oxide as a biomaterial, specifically in hip prostheses. It was concluded that it has excellent biocompatibility, observed in both in vitro and in vivo tests, with no adverse local or systemic reactions and its mechanical properties, which allow for a high safety factor in terms of low sensitivity to stress, further favor flexibility in modular design. They are dependent on the precursors and the process involved in manufacturing the components.

Luthardt et al. (2003) proposed the hypothesis that microcracks and surface flaws induced by machining are responsible for the limited fracture resistance of Y-TZP copings. For this purpose, Y-TZP ceramic cylinders with a height of 15 mm (Metoxit, Ag, Thayngen, Switzerland) were used, which were longitudinally sectioned using a diamond disk, where the samples were produced. They were processed by a specific milling unit for each study factor: to evaluate the finish (Precideunt - DCSW, Allschwix - Switzuland), Polishing to evaluate the crack size (Planomiat 408, Blohm GMBIT, Hamburg, Germany) and after the surface treatments, the discs were cleaned with ethanol. The results showed microcracks and flaws in the surface by SEM analysis, thus confirming the study's hypothesis. On the one hand, machining can introduce residual surface compression stresses which can increase the strength of Zirconia ceramics considerably, but on the other hand it can introduce surface flaws which act as stress concentrators. Therefore, alternative machining or non-machining methods should be developed to achieve greater strength and reliability in CAD/CAM fabricated crowns and fixed bridge structures.

Ozcan & Vallittu (2003), in their study, evaluated the effect of current ceramic surface treatment methods on a resin cement with the aim of identifying the best method for treating ceramics before cementation. As a method, thirty-six groups (n = 6) were separated with six ceramics: Finesse, In-Ceram Alumina, In-Ceram Zirconia, IPS Empress II, Procera AllCeram and Experimental Alumina, which were obtained directly from the respective manufacturers. The ceramics were polished with sandpaper no. 1200 and received the following treatments: 1) etching with 9.6% fluoride acid for 90 seconds (except for IPS Empress II - 20 seconds) and silanization with Monobond S; 2) blasting with 110 µm aluminium oxide particles at a pressure of 55.11 psi for 13 seconds at a distance of 10 mm and application of ESPE-Sil silane; 3) Sandblasting with 110 µm salicylic acid-modified aluminum oxide particles at a pressure of 40.60 psi for 13 seconds at a distance of 10 mm and application of ESPE-Sil silane. A layer of Heliobond adhesive was applied and light-cured, after which Variolink II cement was manipulated and applied to the ceramic surface in a matrix with perforations 3.6 mm in diameter and 5 mm high and light-cured for 40 seconds. Half of the samples were stored in water at room temperature for 24 hours and the other half were thermocycled 6000 times from 5 to 55 °C for 30 seconds each. The mechanical shear test was carried out on a universal testing machine at a speed of 1.0 mm/min. The authors concluded that: the bond strength of resin cement to ceramics after surface treatment varied according to the type of ceramic; the findings confirmed that etching with fluoride acid is the method of choice for cementing ceramics containing vitreous matrix with Bis-GMA-based cements; surface roughening with sandblasting before cementation promoted greater bond strength for ceramics with a high alumina content and the values increased more after silicatization; thermocycling decreased the bond strength values in all the surface treatments tested.

Moraes (2004), in his thesis on the physical and chemical properties of zirconium oxide, states that these composites are promising candidates for use as implant materials. In the present work, ten different compositions were analysed in which the content of yttrium-stabilized zirconium (Y-TZP) added to alumina varied from 5% to 80% by weight. X-ray diffraction and the Rietveld method were used to quantify the phases present and assess the extent of the zirconium phase transformation. Observations of the microstructure and determination of the mechanical properties of the sintered materials were carried out. Fracture mechanisms present in these composites are discussed in order to better understand the failures. The materials investigated showed a density in the range of 99.13 % to 99.86 % of the theoretical density, which increased with the zirconium content in the composite. These systems can achieve 93 % higher flexural strength and 29 % higher fracture toughness compared to pure alumina. The fracture mode of the materials investigated was predominantly intergranular, and transgranular fracture was observed for pure alumina and composites with 5% zirconium. The increase in fracture toughness is mainly related to the greater density and homogeneity of the microstructure and was proportional to the amount of tetragonal zirconium available for transformation, indicating that the mechanism of toughening by transformation and the micro-trenching associated with this transformation plays an important role in these composites. Flexural strength increased with microstructure refinement, being more sensitive to grain size than fracture toughness.

Fragoso et al. (2005) reported that commercially pure titanium (Ticp) has been widely used in the manufacture of cast prosthetic structures due to its favorable properties. However, the mold temperature recommended by the manufacturer has been considered low, causing inadequate castability and poor marginal adaptation of cast crowns. This study evaluated and compared the influence of mold temperature (430°C as a control, 550°C, 670°C) on the marginal discrepancy of Ticp cast crowns. Eight bovine teeth were prepared on a lathe and shaped to produce eight master models. Twenty-four crowns were made in TiCP for three mold temperature groups (n=8): 430°C (as a control), 550°C and 670°C. The marginal gap between the crown and the bovine tooth was observed under a measuring microscope (50X). The marginal adaptation values of the cast crowns were subjected to the Kruskal-Wallis test (P=0.03). The group cast at 550°C (95.0 mm) showed significantly better marginal adaptation than the crowns from the 430°C (203.4 mm) and 670°C (213.8 mm) groups. Better marginal fit was observed for TiCP cast crowns with a mold temperature of 550°C, differing from the manufacturer's recommended temperature of 430°C.

Tsuchimoto et al. (2006) evaluated pretreatment due to the widespread use of titanium for implants in aesthetic sites and the preference for using aesthetic restorative materials such as resin and ceramics. The bonding system for these restorations requires pre-treatment of the titanium surface in order to promote better adhesion of the cement to the substrate, through chemical and mechanical action. To this end, ten 10 mm by 3 mm thick Ti plates were finished and polished, followed by ultrasonic cleaning in ethanol for 5 minutes and immersed in two different solutions of hydrochloric acid (HCl) at concentrations of 0.1 and 1N and a 37% fluoride acid for 5 minutes at room temperature. As a control, additional plates were left untreated after cleaning as above. All treated and untreated plates were rinsed with distilled water for 10 seconds and dried for 5 minutes in oil-free air. Stainless steel rods 7 mm in diameter and 20 mm long were cemented onto the Ti surfaces using Panâvia F cement (Kuraray, Tokyo, Japan) according to the manufacturer's instructions. They were then left to rest for 15 minutes and then stored in water at 37°C for twenty-four hours. Afterwards, the samples were thermocycled for 20,000 cycles and then subjected to a tensile strength test. The data was analyzed by analysis of variance (ANOVA). SEM analysis showed a higher percentage of mixed failures, and the strength values were higher in the non-thermocyclable samples. Therefore, this study sought to develop a simple and safe method of improving the performance of adhesive cementation and to conclude that HCl can be used effectively to improve the adhesive performance of resin to Ti, when it is applied at a concentration of 1N and combined with other methods of micro-mechanical treatment that can further improve the bond.

Matinlinna et al. (2006a) evaluated the adhesive performance of three trialcoxysilane coupling agents. For this purpose, zirconia ceramic samples in the form of plates (10x10x3mm / Procera-Nobel Biocare) were prepared in twelve groups (n=6) and included in acrylic resin blocks, blasted with aluminium oxide (110 mm, 10 mm, 2x13 seconds), ultrasonically cleaned (10 seconds), silicatized (Rocatec Plus - 3M ESPE + 110 mm, 10 mm, 2x13 seconds), ultrasonically cleaned (10 minutes). Silanization of the three agents according to the manufacturer's instructions. The following agents were used: 3-Methacryloyloxypropyltrimethoxysilane (Sigma - Germany); 3- Acryloyloxypropyltrimethoxysilane (Dow Corning loray - Japan); 3- Isocyanatopropyltriethoxysilane (ABCR - Germany). After silanization, the samples were bonded using experimental Bis GMA resins (Rohm - Germany) and commercial RelyX ARC cement (3M ESPE - USA), according to the manufacturers' instructions. The 6 groups were thermocycled with 6000 cycles between 5 and 55°C in deionized water at 2-second intervals and the other six groups were stored at room temperature for 24 hours before testing in a dissector. The specimens were subjected to a shear strength test using a universal testing machine (Lloyd LRX - UK) and the results were analyzed using a three-way ANOVA analysis of variance, with shear strength as the dependent variable and type of silane and type of storage as independent factors. Tukey's test was used for comparative analysis. In this study, the authors concluded that: the shear bond strength test of the three silanizations varied depending on storage and silane; there was no statistical difference between 3-Methacryloyloxypropyltrimethoxysilane and 3-Acryloyloxypropyltrimethoxysilane; thermocycling decreased bond strength values significantly for Bis GMA resin, but not for RelyX ARC, failures were predominantly adhesive: Isocyanotopropyltriethoxysilane does not promote adhesion to Bis GMA resin or RelyX ARC to silicatized zirconia.

Matinlinna et al. (2006 b) evaluated the adhesive performance of silanes on in vitro conditioned titanium surfaces. 3-Acryloyloxypropyltrimethoxysilane and a mixture of 3-Acryloyloxypropyltrimethoxysilane and 1,2-bis (Triethoxysil) ethane were prepared in 95 vol. % ethanol. A commercial silane 3- Methacryloxypropyltrimethoxysilane was used as a control. The silanes were manipulated and applied, according to the respective manufacturers' instructions, to the surface of the titanium blocks (20x40x1mm) treated with tribo chemical silicatization (Cojet - 3M ESPE). Using a matrix, a dendrimer resin was applied to the surface of the silanized titanium, forming 2 x 4 mm tubes which were then photo-polymerized. The specimens were thermocycled (6000 cycles, 5 and 55°C, 30 seconds apart) and then subjected to a shear strength test on a universal testing machine (1RX1 - UK). The data were analyzed using ANOVA analysis of variance and the type of silane as the dependent variable. Tukey's and Levene's methods were used for comparisons of error variances. Given the limitations of this study, the authors concluded that: the silica content on the titanium surface was 41% and not 48%; the new silane system consisting of a mixture of 1,2-bis (triethoxysilyl) ethane produced better adhesion than the others used; 3-Acryloyloxypropylmethoxysilane can form a more hydrolytically stable siloxane film than the others.

Matinlinna et al. (2006 c) evaluated in vitro the action of five dental silanes as adhesion promoters for resin cements on Ti surfaces treated with silicatization. An available cementation kit with its silane was arbitrarily used for the current evaluation and four other silanes were compared with the kit by measuring the shear bond strength. The hypothesis in this evaluation was that all dental silanes have equal bonding properties. Ti grade 2 veneers measuring 20/40mm were used. They were blasted with aluminum oxide (50µm) in a 300 kpa jet at a distance of 10 mm and perpendicular to the veneer. They were ultrasonically cleaned in ethanol for 10 minutes and the surface silicatized using the

Rocatec system (3M ESPE - EVA). Five groups were made and labeled by the agent used per group, half of which were thermocycled and the other not, each group with eight samples in all. After drying, the respective silanes were applied and left to react for two minutes. The cement was manipulated according to the manufacturer's instructions for 10 seconds and applied to a polyethylene matrix (2 mm in diameter and 4 mm high) and polymerized for 40 seconds in all samples. Half were kept dry for an hour before testing and the other was thermocycled with 6,000 cycles at temperatures ranging from 5 to 55°C with a 30-second immersion time pattern. Shear strength tests were carried out using a universal testing machine (LRX1, L10Y Instruments, UK) and the results obtained were analyzed using a two-way analysis of variance (ANOVA) followed by Tukey's test, which showed that the brand of silane and the types of storage conditions differed statistically significantly ($P < 0.05$) and not significantly ($P < 0.05$).0.05) and there was no interaction between silane and storage conditions ($P=0.725$). The hypothesis defined by the authors cannot be verified: All five silanes do not promote equal bonding. Thermocycling weakens shear strength and silanes with lower pH (4.0 and 4.5) provide a stronger bond than those with higher pH (5.5 and 6.0). It can be concluded that these results do not suggest that any silane can be used for bonding a resin cement to silica-coated titanium.

Sundh & Sjogren (2006), looking at the mechanical properties of Zirconium, carried out a study with the aim of identifying the fracture resistance of Zirconium prefabricated with different stabilizing oxides and amounts of sintering. To this end, four stainless steel master abutments were made, prepared with standardized inclinations, dimensions and ends, and included in silicon moulds, simulating the position of the second premolar and second molar with identical distances, producing two models that were sent to each company, to be produced as TZP and PSZ Magnesium Fixed Partial Denture frameworks, in different companies using CAD/CAM technology and then sintered. The frameworks were covered with feldspathic porcelain by a laboratory technician and cemented to the models with a zinc phosphate cement, according to the technique. The cemented PPFs were stored in water for twenty-four hours at 37°C and then subjected to dynamic loading, 100,000 cycles with 90 loads/min between 0 and 50N. The specimens were loaded to fracture using a universal machine tester (Alewtron TCT 5/10). From the results obtained, it can be concluded that fixed partial denture (FPD) frameworks with $Y\text{-}ZrO2$ and $Mg\text{-}ZrO2$ appear to be interesting alternatives for use as all-ceramic fixed bridge frameworks, but clinical studies with long follow-up times are nevertheless necessary to evaluate the clinical performance of the systems.

Lüthy et al. (2006) aimed to evaluate the shear strength of seven different cements on surfaces blasted with aluminum oxide, before and after thermocycling. To this end, 10 Y-TZP samples were prepared for cementation on metal cylinders. All the Y-TZP samples were blasted with aluminium oxide (110µm) and divided into seven groups according to the cement used (n=30): Ketac (glass ionomer-based); Nexus (ordinary Bis-GMA); Superbond (with 4-Meta principle); Panàvia 21 (with MDP); Panàvia F (with MDP); RelyX Unicem (with functional monomer); and the seventh group was silicatized with Rocatec (3M ESPE, Seefeld, Germany) before cementation with Nexus. Half of the samples were stored for forty-eight hours at 37°C and the other half underwent 10,000 thermocycling cycles between 5-55°C. The shear bond strength test was applied to all species, statistical tests were carried out and flaws were determined by microscopy. The group with the highest bond strength was Panâvia 21 (Kuraray, Osaka, Japan), while the groups with Ketac and Nexus cements had the worst results regardless of thermocycling and showed greater cohesive failures. The Nexus + Rocatec group had significantly increased strength. Before thermocycling: Panâvia 21 > Panâvia F > Superbond = RelyX Unicem. Thermocycling affected the bond strength of all the cements, with Panavia F and 21 having an increase in bond strength, while Superbond had a reduction in shear bond strength. The authors concluded that the cements with MDP obtained the best results due to their bond with metal oxides and the Rocatec system was decisive for Nexus to obtain good results, but it is believed that thermocycling should be carried out for longer periods.

Schneider et al. (2007) carried out a study to determine the tensile strength of dual resin cements on Ticp at 10 minutes and 24 hours after removal of the oxide layer. The preference in this study was to use dual cement because the light used for polymerization does not reach the cement due to the blockage of the metal surface. 120 Ticp discs were made, polished with 320, 400 and 600 grit silicon carbide sandpaper, embedded in plastic cylinders and cast in self-curing acrylic resin. The samples were surface treated with aluminum oxide blasted with 50µm particles for 5 seconds at a distance of 5 mm and 80 psi of pressure. After blasting, they were ultrasonically cleaned for 10 minutes and divided into 4 groups (n=30). Bonding was carried out immediately (groups 1 and 3) and twenty-four hours later in groups 2 and 4. Panâvia F cement (Kuraray, Japan) was used in groups 1 and 2 and RelyX ARC (3M Dental Products, USA) in groups 3 and 4, following the manufacturer's instructions. In groups 1 and 2, a primer containing MDP and VBATDT monomers (Alloy Primer, Kuraray, Japan) was applied to enable bonding with the cement. In groups 3 and 4, a silane agent (Primer Ceramic 3M, USA) was applied for the same purpose. All the samples were bonded and the cements were handled and used according to the manufacturer's instructions. A cylindrical plastic matrix was used to keep the discs centered and aligned in the correct place after applying the cement and light to moderate pressure was applied with the fingers. After curing, the samples were stored in water at 37°C for twenty-four hours. The tensile strength test was carried out on a universal testing machine (Instron Company, MA, USA) and the values recorded in MPA were analyzed by analysis of variance (ANOVA) where P=0.05. To determine the mode of fracture, the samples were observed under a 60X stereoscopic magnifier (Carls Zeiss, Germany) and then observed using an SEM (Heo 435 VP, France). The results obtained showed that both cements obtained tensile strength values with no significant differences (P>0.05) and that they did not show the same failure mode, being adhesive for RelyX ARC and predominantly cohesive for Panâvia F, due to the action of the MDP monomer and its primer, promoting greater wetting.

Wolfart et al. (2007) studied the durability of resin cements on zirconium Y-TZP . Zr Y-TZP disks (6.4 x 3.4 mm) were used as specimens forming six groups (n=20) depending on the etching method and resin cement used. After surface treatment, all samples were cleaned in 96% isopropanol for 3 minutes. Groups: ORG-V - Heliobond + Variolink II, was applied to the original ceramic surface; APW-V - The ceramic surface was cleaned with sodium hydrocarbonate solution spray prior to the application of Heliobond and Variolink II; ABR-V - The ceramic surface was abraded with Al O_{23} , prior to the application of Heliobond and Variolink II; ORG-P - Panavia F was applied to the original ceramic surface supplied by the manufacturer; APW-P - The surface was cleaned with a sodium hydrocarbon solution spray prior to applying Panavia F; ABR-P - Panavia F was applied to the sanded and polished ceramic surface. The groups were divided into two subgroups (n=10). One subgroup was stored in distilled water at 37°C without thermocycling for 3 days and the other was stored under the same conditions for 150 days with thermal cycles of 37,500 at 5° and 55°C and subjected to the tensile strength test. The results for Variolink II ranged from 9[a] to 16 MPA (p<0.05) than for Panavia F ranging from 18.7 - 45.5 MPA. Air abrasion resulted in a significantly higher TBS (p < or = 0.01) than the other two surface conditioning methods. After 150 days of storage, only the samples that had been air abraded and bonded with Panavia F showed higher bond strengths (39.2 MPA), most of the other samples had shifted spontaneously or showed very low bond strengths. It can be concluded that not only cleaning, roughening and surface activation by sandblasting prior to adhesive bonding and the use of resin compounds containing MDP are necessary for a durable bond to densely synthesized zirconium ceramics.

Manicone et al. (2007) through a study aimed at the basic properties and clinical applicability of the use of Zirconium partially stabilized with itrium oxide, reviewed the literature showing an overview of $ZrO2$. Although long-term clinical evaluation is a fundamental requirement, it was concluded that Y-ZrO2 has good reliability for dental use,

Published biological, mechanical and clinical studies seem to indicate that ZrO restorations$_2$ are sufficiently well tolerated and resistant. Ceramic coverage, cementation, aging and wear must be evaluated in order to guide the appropriate use of Zirconium as a prosthetic restoration material, and patient selection and appropriate clinical and technical protocols are imperative in order to obtain good performance from these restorations.

Oyagüe et al. (2009) evaluated the effect of zirconia surface treatment on adhesion strength with different adhesive cements by comparing samples treated with 125µm Al2O3 jet, 50µm Al2O3 jet with silica and no treatment. The three resin cements used in this study were: Calibra, Clearfil Esthetic Cement and RelyX Unicem. Eighteen cylinder-shaped zirconium oxide ceramic blocks (Cercon, Dentsply) were subjected to the appropriate treatments. The ceramic cylinders were duplicated in composite resin (Tetric, Ivoclair Vivadent) using a silicone mold. After the samples had been conditioned, the cements were handled according to the manufacturer's instructions with polymerization lasting 40 seconds and then stored in a laboratory oven for 24 hours at 37°C and 100% relative humidity. The samples were subjected to the micro-tensile test using a universal testing machine (Instron 4411, USA) at a speed of 0.5mm per minute until failure. With the results and data analysis, it was observed that adhesive strength is significantly influenced by the adhesive agent, but not by the surface treatment. The adhesion of Clearfil, which contains MDP, to zirconia was much higher than that of RelyX Unicem and Calibra. The samples treated with an Al2O3 jet (125µm) showed a change in the surface which caused micro retention. Those treated with silica showed a slight surface modification. It should be noted that adhesive agents with MDP seem to be the most suitable for adhesion to zirconium without the need for surface treatment, although this adhesion can be improved by blasting with Al O_{23} . Cements that do not contain MDP, self-adhesive cements and conventional cements have proved to be less effective; however, the durability of these chemical bonds must be assessed.

Aboushelib et al. (2009) evaluated the long-term performance of the bond strength between resin and zirconia using selective etch infiltration (SIE) in combination with new zirconia primers in vitro. The hypothesis proposed was that the different reactions of the primers would produce different values after 90 days of water storage at 37°C. To this end,

40 zirconia disks (19.5mm x 3mm - Procera Zirconia, Sweden) received SIE (Selective Infiltration Etching) treatments and were coated with one of the four new zirconia primers (n=10). The primers used in these studies are: primer 1: 3-Acryloyloxypropyltrimethoxysilane with 95% purity (Gelest, USA); primer 2: 3-Isocyanatopropyltryetoxysilane with 95% purity (ABCR, Germany); primer 3: 3-Styrylethytrimethoxysilane with 95% purity (ABCR, Germany); primer 4: 3-Methacrylloyloxypropyltrimethoxysilane with purity greater than 95% (Dow Corning USA). After applying the primers to all the samples, composite resin disks (Tetric, Ivoclair) were bonded to the zirconium disks using Panâvia F 2.0 cement, according to the manufacturer's instructions. The samples were then cut into sticks and one half was subjected to the micro-tensile test and the other half was stored in natural water for 90 days. The results were subjected to a two-way analysis of variance (ANOVA). Storage in water resulted in a significant decrease ($p<0.001$) in the strength of the resin/zirconia bond. By SEM, the failure that predominated in the group after water storage was interfacial and in the group without, it was cohesive, indicating a decrease in bond strength values. This may be related to two factors such as the hydrolysis effect of water on adhesive joints and the fact that it is characterized by the structural metamorphosis of the monomer initiators which, in the polymerization process, pass through the phases taking on hydrophobic -> hydrophilic -> hydrophobic characteristics. hydrophilic -> hydrophobic as a mechanism of water inhibition in which a small delay in the change to the hydrophobic state may be sufficient to interfere with the bond in the presence of water, leading to an increase in the thickness of the cement and a break in the established bond. In conclusion, the stability of the resin/zirconia bond is directly related to the chemistry of the materials used, including the primers, and further research is needed to develop more hydrophobic compounds that better resist the damaging effect of hydrolysis in order to obtain benefits from the primers tested.

Piascik et al. (2009) in this study aimed to develop and evaluate a practical method for chemically modifying the surface of zirconia ceramics to facilitate viable adhesive bonding using commercially available silanes and resin cements. This technique consists of water vapor deposition of silicon tetrachloride ($SiCl_4$) in which, upon reacting with the substrate surface, active hydroxyl groups are formed on the surface and subsequently form a layer of silicon oxide (SiO) on the substrate surface. Pre-sintered zirconia blocks (14x12x20mm) were obtained from the manufacturer (ZirCAD-Ivoclair) and resin composite blocks (Aelite-Bisco) were manufactured (14x12x20mm). The surfaces of each material were polished and blasted with aluminum oxide (50µm, 0.29 Mpa at 20 seconds) and ultrasonically cleaned for 5 minutes before chemical treatment and bonding. Functionalization on the zirconia surface was carried out using reaction with silicon tetrachloride ($SiCl_4$), reaction with water by vapor deposition using a commercial apparatus (MDV - 100 San Jose - CA), resulting in the deposition of a layer of SiO particles, a by-product of hydrochloric acid gas. The thickness of the film was controlled by the deposition time. For this study, two thicknesses were used (2.6 and 23 mm). After treatment, the ceramic and resin blocks were bonded together using resin cement (C&B, Bisco) and were stored at room temperature for 24 hours and turned into bar specimens for micro traction. Group 1: fluoride acid + silane; Group 2: silane only; Group 3: Cojet + silane; Group 4: 2.6 mm thick SiO + silane; Group 5: 23 mm thick SiO + silane. All the samples were subjected to the micro-tensile test and the results obtained were analyzed by ANOVA analysis of variance, which revealed a significant difference in the mean adhesive strength. Samples with surface treatments exhibited greater adhesive strength. Several types of failure modes were revealed, around 85% of which proved to be mixed mode and cohesive. Therefore, the increased bond strength of surface treated zirconia/composite can be derived from the optimization of SiO thickness and roughness combination allowing a strong bonding of these high strength dental ceramics in a new range of applications. It is concluded that this approach can improve the adhesion of resin to zirconia using traditional silane and cementation techniques.

Almeida et al. (2010), taking into account the effectiveness of surface treatment in promoting a strong bond strength of resin cements to metals, they can contribute significantly to the long life of metal-ceramic restorations. This study evaluated the effect of surface treatment on the bonding of a resin cement to titanium. Ninety discs were cast in Ticp and divided into 3 groups (n=30), which received the following blasting conditions: 1) 50μm Al O_{23} particles; 2) 30μm silica-modified Al O_{23} particles (Cojet Sant); 3) 110μm silica-modified Al2O3 particles (Rocatec). For each blasting condition, the following post-blasting treatments were used (n=10): 1) None; 2) Silane RelyX Ceramic Primer. RelyX ARC resin cement was applied to the TiCP surface. The specimens were thermocycled before testing. The fracture mode was also determined. The best combination was Rocatec with silane. All groups showed 100% adhesive failure.

Qeblawi et al. (2010) evaluated the effect of mechanical treatment of Y- PSZ on its flexural strength and analyzed the effect of chemical treatment on the bond strength with resin cement. The study included 74 sintered Zr bars which were divided into 4 groups according to surface treatment: 1) control group; 2) Al2O3 blasting - 50μm; 3) silicatization using 30µm particles (Cojet); 4) fine grinding (by hand). The bars were stored for 24 hours before the flexural strength values were checked. Another 32 cut bars formed a total of 192 Y-PSZ rods, which were divided into 4 groups (n=48) according to the mechanical treatments and subdivided into 4 new groups (n=12) according to the chemical treatment: 1) Control; 2) HF 4.5% for 3 minutes + Silane 3-MPS; 3) Silane 3-MPS only; 4) Zirconia Primer. All the samples were cemented using Multilink cement on human teeth and the shear strength test was applied. The 5 groups were subjected to storage at room temperature for 90 days and 20,000 thermocycling cycles between 5° and 55°C. The results obtained from the studies were that sandblasting and fine grinding significantly increased flexural strength. All the mechanical treatments resulted in an increase in bond strength and all the chemical treatments provided an increase in shear strength. Among the groups, the silicatization + silane combination obtained the highest shear bond strength. According to the mechanical treatments, in the group that was blasted with Al $_{23}$ /silane/primer-MDP increased resistance, while acid etching had very little influence. When silicatization was carried out, the high strength values were due to the need to apply silane afterwards to obtain a chemical bond with the impregnated silica. When milling was carried out, the MDP primer and acid/silane conditioning resulted in the highest shear strength. The groups that underwent artificial ageing had a durable bond when it is preceded by a surface treatment that provides mechanical retention.

Shaim & Kern (2010) evaluated the effect of air-abrasion surface treatment on the retention of CAD/CAM zirconia crowns (Cerec 3 CAD/CAM, Vita In Ceram, Germany) cemented with three different types of cement. In addition, the influence of artificial ageing, a masticatory simulator and thermal cycling were tested. The samples were randomly distributed into three groups of 32 samples (n=32), referring to the three cements used. Half of the crowns received surface treatment with air-abrasion and ultrasonic washing for 5 minutes in ethanol solution. For cementation, all the manufacturer's instructions were followed and the cements were standardized under a pressure of 20N for 10 minutes: Zinc phosphate cement (Hoffman), glass ionomer cement (Ketac Cem) and resin cement (Panàvia 21).

Subgroups of 8 samples were formed and stored for 3 days at 37°C in water; for 150 days at 37°C in 37,500 thermal cycles (5°-55°C) and 300,000 dynamic load cycles with 5 kilos in a masticatory simulator. All the samples were tested for bond strength on a universal testing machine and then analyzed using ANOVA, three-way analysis of variance and Tukey's test. The average strength values were 2.8 to 7.1 MPa after 3 days and 1.6 to 6.1

MPa after artificial ageing. Sandblasting resulted in greater crown retention ($p<0.001$), while artificial ageing reduced retention ($p=0.017$). In addition, resin cement had a significant influence on retention, increasing it ($p<0.001$). With the results obtained, the following conclusions were made: resin cement with MDP achieved greater retention than conventional cements; Al blasting O_{23} improved retention regardless of the cement; long-term artificial ageing with mechanical loading decreased crown retention, regardless of the cement used.

Mirmohammadi et al. (2010) compared the adhesion values and rank order of three resin cements using the micro tensile (TBS) and micro shear (SBS) tests. Zirconia discs (11.8mmx3mm) were polished and blasted with 50µm aluminum oxide particles at a pressure of 0.35 Mpa and a distance of 1 cm, after which they were cleaned in an ultrasonic tank with distilled water for 10 minutes. Filtek 250 composite resin discs (11.8mmx3mm) were made and cemented to the ceramic discs using three different cements (Panâvia F 2.0 - Kuraray, RelyX Unicem - 3M ESPE and Multilink Automix - Ivoclair - Vivadent). The blocks were cut and submitted to the micro traction test (n=10). For the micro shear test, zirconia disks (22 mm x 0.8 mm) and Filtek 250 composite resin disks (0.9 m x 0.7 mm) were made. The same surface treatment and cementation protocol used for the micro-tensile test was used. The specimens were then tested using the shear test (n=10). The results were subjected to two-way ANOVA statistical analysis. There was a statistically significant difference in bond strength values between the cements tested and also between the evaluation methods used. The micro traction test reported a significant difference in adhesive strength values, while the micro shear test detected no difference. For the micro-tensile test, Panâvia F (32.5 +- 1.7 Mpa) showed a statistically significant difference from the other resin cements, RelyX Unicem (24.2 +- 2.7) and Multilink showed cohesive failures of the resin cement, while RelyX Unicem showed predominant adhesive failures. Based on this study, the authors concluded that the micro-tensile test was able to detect differences in bond strength between the three phosphate monomers contained in the structures of zirconia resin cements, while the micro-shear test was unable to detect such differences.

Yun et al. (2010) carried out a study to evaluate the effect of blasting and metal primers on the shear strength of three commercial cements for cementing Y-TZP zirconia ceramics. One hundred and twenty Y-TZP ceramic cylinders were made and placed in polytetrafluoroethylene molds. The specimens were divided into 12 groups (n=10) according to the surface treatment. Different types of treatment were used on the zirconia ceramic. Three resin cements with their respective metallic primers were used (Alloy Primer - Panâvia F 2.0; V-Primer - Superbond C&B; Metalite - Mbond), together with the use of aluminum oxide blasting, to cement the specimens to the zirconia ceramic. After thermocycling (5000 cycles), the specimens were subjected to a shear test and the best adhesive values were obtained when ceramic primers were used in conjunction with aluminum oxide blasting (90µm, 10 mm, 3.8 bar, 15 seconds). The conclusion of this work, based on the results of this experiment, showed that the use of metal primers and resin cements alone are not enough to achieve a lasting bond with Y-TZP ceramic, so it is necessary to sandblast the surface to improve adhesion levels.

Yang et al. (2010) evaluated the influence of surface conditioning parameters with and without sandblasting, and sandblasting at pressures of 0.05 Mpa and 0.25 Mpa combined with a resin cement, checking them with resistance tests after storage in water and thermal cycling. Zirconium oxide ceramic disks (Cercon, Germany) were made and polished with 600 grit sandpaper. Three surface conditions were used: No blasting; blasting with Al O_{23} particles, 50µm, 0.25 Mpa at a distance of 10 mm per second. The samples were then ultrasonically cleaned in ethanol. 96% ethanol for 2 minutes. They were air-dried and applied with Metal/Zirconia Primer (MZP, Ivoclair); Alloy Primer (Kuraray, Japan); Clearfil/Ceramic Primer (Kuraray, Japan), used according to the manufacturer's instructions. Cements were made in the form of tubes using RelyX Unicem cement (3M ESPE), according to the manufacturer's instructions. They were then stored in water for 3 and 150 days at 37°C and subjected to 37,500 thermal cycles from 5° to 55°C, after which the strength test was carried out on a testing machine (Zwick, Germany). The samples were analyzed using the Wilcoxon test for multiple testing at α=5%. The hypothesis that there is no influence of surface treatment with primers on the bond with Zr in the long term, and that the reduction in air pressure associated with the primers in this study had no influence on the bond with the ceramic had to be rejected. In conclusion, when using composite resin containing MDP in combination with primers containing MDP, a long-term bond with Zr ceramic is provided and without sandblasting, no long-term bond was achieved regardless of the use of primers.

Attia & Kern (2011) carried out a laboratory study in which their aim was to evaluate the influence of surface conditioning, new ceramic primers and cleaning methods on the bond strength and tensile strength of resin to zirconia ceramic (E-max - ZirCAD) and their interactions. 96 zirconia disks were divided into six groups (n=16) according to the conditioned surface, cleaning method and ceramic primers. After preparing the discs for cementation, transparent plastic tubes with an internal diameter of 3.2 mm were made, filled with composite resin and polymerized. Next, a dual adhesive cement (Multilink automix) was used to bond the resin tubes to the discs and an alignment device was used under a load of 750 gr and polymerized. Each main group was divided into two subgroups (n=8). Eight samples were stored in the distilled water bath at 37°C for three days without thermocycling, while the other eight samples were stored for thirty days in the same water bath at 37°C interrupted by thermal cycles between 5 and 55°C in distilled water with a dwell time of 30 seconds (Willytec, Germany) for 7,500 cycles. The samples were subjected to a universal test on a machine (Zwick 2010, Germany) for the tensile bond strength test. The results obtained showed no significant difference between the groups tested, regardless of the factors. Within the limitations of this study, it was concluded that the method of cleaning after surface conditioning had no significant effect on the bond strength of the resin to zirconia after thirty days' storage of the specimens and after artificial ageing, a universal primer (Monobond plus) containing a silane and a phosphate monomer was able to promote an improvement in the bonding of the resin to the silica-coated zirconium ceramic, compared to the use of a conventional silane.

Kim et al. (2011) investigated the shear bond strength of various cements (Fuji I, Ketac Cem Easymix, Fuji Plus, RelyX Luting, Principle, Lonotite, Panâvia F 2.0 and RelyX Unicem). 32 cylinder-shaped zirconia ceramic disks (20 mm in diameter and 1.5 mm thick) (LAVA, 3M ESPE, Germany) were prepared according to the manufacturer's instructions. The disks were placed in PVA tubes (25.4 mm in diameter and 19.0 mm high) wrapped in acrylic resin so that the surface to be used for cement adhesion was uncovered. A matrix was made to fit over the cylinder, with a central hole measuring 3.17mm and 1.00mm high where the cement would be inserted and adhered to the zirconia surface. The cements were manipulated and inserted into the hole in the matrix and polymerized according to the manufacturer's instructions on the zirconia, which had previously been treated with sandblasting (Al O_{23} , 110 mm to 10 mm at a pressure of 0.25 Mpa for 13 seconds), after which they were ultrasonically cleaned with isopropyl alcohol for 3 minutes. All the samples were stored in water at 37°C for 48 hours. Half of the specimens in each group were thermocycled before the shear test. A testing machine (Instron Inc, USA) was used for the test, after which the samples were examined under an optical microscope (SMZ800) to determine the mode of fracture. Surface roughness and surface energy parameters were evaluated using the contact angle method. After the test, the samples were subjected to statistical analysis. Panavia F 2.0 and Principle cements showed the highest adhesion values with no significant changes before and after thermocycling.

Adhesive rupture occurred in all the samples that failed. It can therefore be concluded that surface energy parameters should be taken into account when evaluating cement adhesive properties with zirconia ceramics.

Behr et al. (2011) investigated the shear bond strength (SBS) and tensile strength of the zirconia/resin interface using different bonding concepts with resin cements. To do this, CoCr (Chrome/Cobalt) cylinders measuring 5 mm in diameter and 3 mm in height were bonded to coplanar zirconia specimens (Degudent, Hanau, G) 2 mm thick, 20 mm long and 10 mm wide. The surfaces of the parts to be used for bonding were blasted with Al O_{23} (110µm, 10 seconds at 0.28Mpa), and the CoCr cylinders were applied a Metal Primer (GC, Tokyo). The bonding concepts consisted of the application of a silane coupling agent, silica tribological coating (Rocatec system), resin cements and primers containing phosphone, monophosphate and diphosphate, and a combination of primer with the silica arrangement. All the cements were handled according to the manufacturer's instructions and applied to the surfaces and bonded under a pressure of 1 kg for 20 seconds. The lateral surfaces of the cementing agents were light-cured and stored in distilled water at 37°C for 5 minutes. The SBS and TBS tests were determined after 24 hours and 90 days of storage in distilled water at 37°C as well as 12,000 thermal cycles (5° / 55°C, 2 minutes, 17 days). The predominant mode of failure was adhesive failure on the ceramic surface. Therefore, the results obtained conclude that to date no bonding concept can offer a strong and reliable long-term bond between resins and zirconia that can withstand oral loading conditions.

Thompson et al. (2011) reported in their literature review that zirconium oxide-based ceramics have become a topic of great interest in the field of dental prostheses and implants. One problem with the clinical use of zirconia components is the difficulty of achieving adequate adhesion with synthetic substrates or natural tissues. Traditional adhesive techniques used with silica-based ceramics do not work effectively with zirconia. He said that various technologies are being used clinically to solve this problem, and other approaches are being investigated. Most focus on modifying the inert surface of high-strength ceramics. The ability to chemically functionalize the zirconia surface appears to be critical in obtaining an adhesive bond. This review focused on currently available approaches as well as new advanced technologies to solve this problem, concluding that although the science and technology applied to adhesion has improved, there is still much to be learned to make this behavior predictable for clinical use.

Smith et al. (2011) compared the bond between composite and zirconia using the usual surface conditioning treatments and a new technique that combines water vapor with silicon tetrachloride to form a silicate layer on the ceramic surface. The test groups were: 1) Control: vitreous ceramic treated with 5% fluoride acid + silane; 2) Zirconia treated with silicatization with 30mm particles + silane; 3) Application of metal/zirconia primer on the zirconia; 4) Layer of silica deposited varying respectively from 3.7mm, 5.8mm and 30.4mm + silane. Resin blocks were cemented to the ceramic blocks with Clearfil cement and then the micro-tensile test was carried out after storage for twenty-four hours (baseline) and after 1, 3 and 6 months. SEM analysis showed that the failures were all adhesive. Statistical tests showed that at baseline the highest values belonged to groups 1, 2 and 4. After the first month, bonding increased in all groups (except group 5), especially in the control group. At three months, groups 1, 2 and 4 maintained good results and at six months only group 2 was statistically similar to group 1. The authors therefore concluded that the arrangement of the silica vapor layer requires further studies that include the effects of aging, since the only group comparable in terms of durable bonding to porcelain was the one treated with silicatization/silane.

Kawai et al. (2012) focused in this study on cyclic impact and shear loading on the bond strength of three resin cements to zirconia by the shear bond strength test. Two disks of different sizes (10x10x20mm and 10x10x10mm) of Y-TZP were prepared (n=81), and they were planed and polished (220, 400 and 600) with silicon carbide disks and surface treated with the Rocatec system (3M ESPE) for 13 seconds at 0,25 Mpa, cleaned with air for 5 seconds, coated with a layer of Espe-Sil silane (3M ESPE) and left to dry for 5 minutes before applying the cement. The following cements were used: Superbond C and B (Sun Medical) (SB); Panâvia Fluoro Cement (Kuraray) (PF) and resin-reinforced glass ionomer cement (Fuji Lining) (IVR). After handling and applying the cements according to the manufacturer's instructions, the samples were subjected to a pressure of 15 kg for 15 minutes in order to standardize the application of cementation pressure. The samples were subsequently subjected to three storage conditions: 106 compression cyclic impact load (CL), 106 shear cyclic impact load and no load (control) and stored in distilled water at 37°C with a mechanical fatigue (FM) device. The samples were subjected to the shear strength test at a speed of 0.5mm/minute until failure occurred. From the results, bond strengths in PF plus control and PF plus CL were significantly higher than with SB and FM. There was no significant difference between IVR and CL (p>0.05) with SB and FM. The bond strength of resin-modified glass ionomer (FL) was significantly lower than with PF and SB and all samples showed cohesive failures. Within the limitations of this study, the following was concluded: a) PF cement containing MDP in combination with Rocatec system treatment produced a higher bond strength than SB and FM; b) there was no difference in bond strength between the cements used after 10^6 thermocycling cycles; c) after tribochemical zirconium treatment, the cements survived more than 10^6 cycles of 10 kg shear and compression impact loading.

Lung & Matinlinna (2012) reviewed the literature to give an overview of the aspects of silane coupling agents and surface conditioning in dentistry. Silane coupling agents are used as adhesion promoters and are effective in cementing the adhesion between the resin and the silica-based ceramic. They are effective for bonding to dental restorative materials that do not contain silica. Surface treatment on silica-free ceramics improves adhesion with silica coating. This current overview will focus on silane coupling agents and their properties, limitations in promoting adhesion and clinical problems with the use of silanes. Various surface conditioning methods are being used clinically to improve adhesion in resin composites for silica-free restorative materials. The clinical problem with using silanes to promote adhesion is that they degrade over time in the oral environment. Silane agents are not ideal because they meet the minimum requirements for adhesion to composite resin and it is important to evolve the silane/surface treatment ratio to address bond durability. Concluding that silanes play a critical role as mediators to meet the clinical requirements of bond durability; that surface conditioning and silanization are a standard laboratory protocol in dental restorations and repairs; the hydrolytic stability of siloxane bonding formed from silane agents with composite resins and dental restorative materials is contemplated; silane agents have shown recent applications in biomedicine justifying their special role in dentistry and that some may support the idea that silanes will play a leading role in biomaterials science, as there is already work showing their increase in durability and longevity.

Belo et al. (2013) observed that yttria-stabilized polycrystalline tetragonal zirconia (Y-TZP) has been widely used in dentistry as an infrastructure material for crowns and fixed partial dentures due to its mechanical characteristics such as high strength and fracture toughness. The aim of this literature review was to find evidence from *in vitro* and *in vivo* studies regarding the mechanical behavior, adhesion and clinical longevity of fixed prostheses made with Y-TZP IE. Articles were retrieved from the *Medline/Pubmed* online database using the following combinations of keywords: yttria-stabilized tetragonal zirconia ("Y-TZP"), adhesion ("bonding"), mechanical properties ("mechanical properties"), clinical studies ("long-term clinical trials"), longevity ("longevity"). The search covered the years 1990 to 2012. According to the literature, Y-TZP has higher mechanical properties than other dental ceramics due to a toughening mechanism associated with crystalline phase transformation. Furthermore, silicatization associated with silanization has been indicated as the most suitable surface treatment for adhesive cementation of Y-TZP, in addition to the use of a resin cement containing phosphate monomers. In clinical studies, Y-TZP has shown high success rates as single crowns and fixed partial bridges. Although the mechanical and bonding behavior of Y-TZP is not completely clear, studies show promising results in relation to the clinical application of this material.

Gomes et al. (2013) evaluated the granulometry of aluminum oxide blasting, two cementation systems and the composition of the resin cement on the surface of zirconia by micro-tensile strength. Forty zirconia blocks (Cercon, Dentsply) were polished and randomly treated as follows: Group 1 (MT): No treatment; Group 2 (APA I): Sandblasting (Cobra, Reufort) using 25mm particles of Al O_{23} ; Group 3 (APA II): 50mm of Al O_{23} ; Group 4 (APA III): 110mm of Al2O3. Ceramic blocks were duplicated in composite resin. The samples from each group were randomly divided into two subgroups, depending on the type of cement used, for bonding the resin disks to the surface of the pre-treated zirconia. Subgroup 1 (PAN) Clearfil Ceramic Primer + Panâvia F: dual self-etching resin cement with fluoride release; Subgroup 2 (BIF) Bifix SE (VOCO): Self-adhesive cement. After 24 hours, the samples were cut into sticks. Microtensile strength values were obtained using a universal testing machine (0.5mm/minute). Failure modes were recorded and the interface morphology evaluated by SEM. Two-way ANOVA analysis of variance, Students-Newman-Kews test and stepwise linear regression analysis were performed with MTBS ($p<0.05$). Despite the grain size of the blast, the PAN subgroup linked to abrasion-treated surfaces achieved the highest MTBS index and often showed mixed failures. The BIF subgroup did not register significant differences in MTBS, but depending on the etching method showed higher rates of premature and adhesive failures. The null hypothesis of this study was rejected, which states that neither the particle size nor the presence of MDP in the composition of the materials would influence the bond strength of the cement/zirconia interface. In conclusion, the cementing system containing MDP seems to be the most suitable method for bonding to zirconia oxide ceramics, especially after blasting, regardless of particle size.

Miyasaki et al. (2013), looking at the current situation of Zr restorations, carried out a literature review with clinical data from 2010, which reviewed clinical evaluation of Zr restorations, surface finish of Zr restorations and wear of antagonist enamel, bonding between Zr and veneering ceramics, resin-based cementing agents and CAD/CAM fixed dental prosthesis systems. In this study, the most frequent complication with Zr-based fixed dental prostheses was delamination of the veneering porcelain, which is affected by many factors, and the bonding mechanism between the two materials remains unknown. Silicatization of the internal surface of the Zr structure associated with primers is the most reliable cementation system and the high hardness of Y-TZP is more than double that of porcelain, raising concerns. It was also shown that highly polished Y-TZP produced less wear on the antagonist.

Amaral et al. (2014) investigated the potential of new zirconia adhesives and universal adhesives for surface-treated zirconia substrates. To this end, zirconium oxide bars (3.0mm x 3.0mm x 9.0mm) were fabricated and treated as follows: no treatment (C); blasting with 35μm alumina particles (S); air abrasion with 30μm silica particles using one of two systems (Rocatec or SilJet); glazing (G). Groups C and S were subsequently treated with one of the following primers or adhesives: ZP (ZPrime Plus), AZ (AZ Primer); MP (Monobond Plus); SU (ScotchBond Universal) and; EA (an Experimental Adhesive). The Rocatec and SilJet groups were silanized before cementation. Group G samples were etched and silanized. Bars were cemented (Multilink) onto silicate ceramic bars (3.0mm x 3.0mm x 9.0mm) at 90^0 angles, thermocycled (2,500 cycles, 5-55^0 C, 30 s dwell time) and tested for tensile strength. Failure analysis was carried out on fractured specimens to measure the bond area and crack origin. Samples from group C did not survive thermocycling, while CMP, CSU and CEA groups survived thermocycling but yielded low bond strength values. All primers showed better bonding performance after air abrasion with Al particles O_{23} . SilJet was similar to Rocatec, both showing the best bond strength results, along with SMP, SSU and CEA. G promoted intermediate bond strength values. The failure mode was predominantly adhesive on the zirconia surface combined with cementing agent cohesion. From the results obtained and analyzed, it was concluded that universal adhesives (MP, SU, EA) can be a considerable alternative for bonding to zirconia, but surface treatment is still necessary beforehand. Sandblasting with silica particles followed by silane application also showed high bond strength values.

Cvikl et al. (2014) aimed to determine the impact of long-term storage on the adhesion between titanium and zirconia with resin cement. Grade 5 titanium blocks (10mm x 4mm x 4mm) and sintered zirconia discs (3mm x 2mm) were used. All samples were blasted with aluminum oxide (110mm, 10mm, 3bar). The zirconium disks were bonded to the titanium blocks, according to the manufacturer's specifications, with four cements: Panavia F 2.0; GC G-CEM; RelyX Unicem and Smart Cem 2. After adhesive bonding, the specimens were divided into 5 groups (n=5) for different storage conditions: water bath for 24 hours at 370^0 C; water bath for 16 days at 370^0 C; water bath for 150 days at 370^0 C and 6,000 thermocycling cycles at 50^0 C to 550^0 C. Afterwards, all the specimens were tested for shear strength. From the results obtained, long-term storage and thermal cycling differentially affected the bonding of the resin cement.

Inokoshi et al. (2014) reported that zirconium oxide ceramics can no longer be considered non-binding to dental tissue. In the literature, a growing number of studies, in fact, report on the bonding efficiency of different cementation techniques to zirconia. This study has reported on general trends in zirconia bonding by systematically collecting zirconia bond strength data. A search of PubMed and EMBASE revealed 1,371 bond strength tests reported in 144 articles. A shear strength protocol was used most frequently, revealed significantly lower bond levels and was less discriminating than the other test methods. With regard to the cementing technique, the combination of mechanical and chemical pre-treatment seemed particularly crucial to obtain a durable bond to the zirconia. The choice of cement was not revealed as a determining factor after the ageing conditions, as long as the composite cement was used. With regard to the test protocol, a tensile test appeared to be more discriminating, particularly when combined with "water storage" ageing.

Mosele & Borba (2014) state that acid-resistant ceramics such as tetragonal zirconia partially stabilized with yttrium (Y-TZP) can have their bond strength to resin cement improved by abrasion through particle blasting. However, there is no standardization of the parameters used in blast treatment, which can negatively affect the mechanical behaviour of Y-TZP. The aim of this study was to find out, through a literature review, which blasting protocols are used and which protocol results in the best bond strength values to the resin cement and the least degradation of the mechanical properties of Y-TZP. The research strategy involved a search for articles in the Medline/Pubmed online database, from 2003 to 2013, using the keywords: Zirconium, Bond strength, Sandblasting, Mechanical Strength. Twenty-five articles were selected which met the inclusion criteria. The most commonly used particle size was 50 μm for aluminum oxide particles and 110 μm for silica-coated aluminum oxide particles. According to the studies, particle size and blasting time do not influence bond strength values. However, the larger particle size and the type of particle (aluminum oxide) negatively affect the mechanical strength of Y-TZP. There is still controversy about the effect of pressure on the bond strength and mechanical strength of Y-TZP. The use of very low pressures can affect adhesion values. The distance between the blasting tip and the ceramic surface and the time varied between 7 and 30 mm and 5 and 90 s, respectively. It can be concluded that some parameters of the blasting protocol are not yet well defined. Even so, the results of the studies seem to corroborate the recommendation to use small particles and low pressures to achieve the best adhesion results without compromising the mechanical strength of the material.

Papia et al. (2014) defined the following objectives for this systematic literature review: (a) to make an inventory of existing methods for achieving bondable surfaces on zirconium oxide ceramics and (b) to evaluate which methods can provide sufficient bond strength. Current literature studies in vitro bond strength obtained with different surface treatments on zirconium oxide ceramics in combination with adhesive cement systems. It was selected from PubMed and systematically analyzed, complete with reference tracking. The total number of publications included was 127 studies, 23 of which were used for objective b. Surface treatments are divided into seven main groups: as-produced, grinding/polishing, particle blasting, surface coating, laser treatment, acid treatment and primer treatment. There are wide variations, making it difficult to compare the studies. A surface produced from a zirconium oxide ceramic needs to be treated to obtain a durable bond strength. Abrasive surface treatment and/or silicatization as a primary treatment can provide sufficient bond strength for this ceramic. This conclusion, however, needs to be confirmed by clinical studies. There is no universal surface treatment. The specific material to be cemented and the adhesive cement system to be used must be considered.

Souza et al. (2014) stated that a strong and stable bond between the resin cement and the zirconium oxide ceramic restoration is fundamental for longevity, but no technique has been established to provide such a bond when the material is zirconia. The aim of this study was to evaluate the effect of different materials containing 10-methacryloyloxydecyl dihydrogen phosphate (MDP) on the bond strength to zirconium oxide ceramic (Y-TZP). Forty Y-TZP disks (Lava) were cemented to substrates (8 groups, n = 5) with and without the prior application of an experimental primer (MDP); an MDP adhesive (Clearfil S3 Bond Plus or Scotchbond Universal) with an MDP (Clearfil AS); a non-MDP luting resin (RelyX Ultimate). The samples were cut, stored in distilled water and subjected to the microtensile test at 48 hours and again at 6 months after the cementation procedures. The data was analyzed by 4-way ANOVA and Tukey's test. Failure modes were classified with a stereomicroscope and the treated surfaces were analyzed with energy dispersive X-ray spectroscopy. Both adhesive and time significantly affected bond strength. The interaction of either factor was not significant. The use of an adhesive containing MDP and a shorter storage time were associated with greater bond strength. They concluded that the application of an MDP-based adhesive can improve the bond strength of cement with zirconium oxide ceramic. However, the bond strength for all groups did not remain stable over 6 months.

Ahn et al. (2015) carried out this study to evaluate the effects of different phosphate-containing monomers on the shear strength between tetragonal zirconia polycrystal ceramic (Y-TZP) and self-adhesive resin cement containing MDP. In this study, the surfaces of the ceramics were made and divided into six groups (n = 10). The specimens were grouped according to the resin cement used and the surface treatment method. The three treatment groups without sandblasting were subdivided: with Metal / Zirconia Primer (Vivadent Ivoclar, Schaan, Liecht-Enstein), Z-PRIME Plus (BISCO, Schaumburg, USA) and without any priming agent treatment. The remaining three groups were treated by blasting Al O_{23} with granules of 50 µm in size at a distance of 10 mm and 3.5 bar for 15 s, with Metal / Zirconia Primer (Vivadent Ivoclar, Schaan, Liecht- Enstein), Z-PRIME Plus (BISCO, Schaumburg, USA) and without any priming agent treatment. They were then bonded to the zirconia surface using self-adhesive resin cement (Clearfil SA Luting, Kuraray, Kurashiki, Okayama, Japan) and light-cured. After thermocycling, a shear strength test was carried out. The surfaces of the Y-TZP samples were analyzed using a scanning electron microscope. The bond strength values were statistically analyzed. It was concluded that: the application of self-adhesive resin cement containing MDP without pre-treatment was not sufficient to improve the bond strength to an untreated Y-TZP surface; the application of an initiating agent containing MDP appears to be a reliable method for increasing the bond strength between Y-TZP ceramic and self-adhesive resin containing MDP.

Della Bona et al. (2015) conducted a literature review, analyzing published studies on zirconium oxide-based ceramics and their current applicability in dentistry. Among all dental ceramics, zirconia is in evidence as a dental biomaterial and is the material of choice in contemporary restorative dentistry. Zirconia has been applied as a structural material for dental bridges, crowns, inserts, and implants, mainly because of its biocompatibility, high fracture toughness, and radiopacity. However, the clinical success of restorative dentistry has to consider adhesion to different substrates, which offers a great challenge for research and development. This study characterizes zirconia as a dental biomaterial, presenting the current consensus and the challenges of its dental applications. Considering in vitro studies and clinical trials, the two most popular clinical strategies for resin bonding acid-resistant ceramic restorations are: improving mechanical retention with a blasting system using alumina particles associated with a chemical bonding mechanism, using an adhesive/cement system containing ceramic initiators, such as phosphate-based monomers, e.g. MDP; improving mechanical retention with a sandblasting system using silica-coated alumina particles to introduce a layer of silica onto the uneven ceramic surface, followed by a silane coupling agent, which promotes a chemical bond with any resin-based adhesive/cement system. In general, the most common causes of structural defects in ceramics are fractures initiated in the connector area of fixed partial dentures (FPD) and delamination of the porcelain covering. The mode of failure is an important aspect of bond strength testing, but is not commonly reported. Detailed inspection of the fractured surface can indicate the mode of failure and is important for understanding and predicting the reliability of the bond interface, reducing the risk of errors in data interpretation. This review has shown that reasoning in adhesion to zirconia ceramics should develop the fundamental basis for understanding the clinical performance of zirconia-based adhesive restorations, the possible causes of failure, and the principles for improving the adhesion mechanisms of resin-based composites bonded to zirconia.

Long et al. (2015) evaluated the in vitro effect of titanium surface treatment with a polydimethylsiloxane coating on the bond strength of a composite resin cement to titanium. The titanium samples (40 to 30 mm) were divided into 4 groups (n = 12). A control group was surface treated by sandblasting with silica-coated aluminum oxide at a constant pressure of 300 kPa for 15s / 1cm2. For the other three groups, a polydimethylsiloxane silicate silicone grease was applied to the surface without blasting. The samples were subjected to heat treatment at temperatures of 800^0 C, 1000^0 C and 11000 C for 2h. A silane coupling agent was then applied and a resin compound was bonded using the polyethylene mold. The samples were subjected to three different conditions: dry storage, water storage in deionized water at 37°C for 30 days and thermocycling for 6000 cycles between 5.0 and 55.0°C. The shear bond strengths of all test groups were determined using a universal testing machine. The data was analyzed by two-way ANOVA and Tukey's test. The results showed that there was a significant difference for different surface treatments and different storage conditions in the average shear strength test forces. The analysis showed that there was a change in the elemental composition of the titanium surface after heat treatment of the coating. It was concluded that the surface treatment of titanium with a polydimethylsiloxane coating at 1000 1C and 1100 1C curing provides sufficient bonding for resin cement for clinical services.

Ozcan & Bernasconi (2015) report that there is currently no consensus on the best adhesion protocol for zirconia used in dentistry, this is particularly important for restorations where mechanical retention is poor. This systematic review analyzed the adhesion potential of resin and glass ionomer cements to zirconia in order to highlight the possible dominant factors affecting the results of bond strength to this substrate. Original scientific documents on adhesion to zirconia published in the MEDLINE (PubMed) database between 01/01/1995 and 01/06/2011 were included in this systematic review. The following MeSH terms, search terms and their combinations were used: "Dental bonding", "Zirconium", "Zirconia", "Y-TZP", "Y-TZP ceramic", "Materials testing/methods", "Testing", "Cement" and "Resin bonding". Two reviewers screened and abstracted the data. Descriptive statistics were performed and the frequencies of the parameters studied, means, standard deviations, confidence intervals (95% CI, uncorrected and corrected), medians and interquartile ranges (IQR) were calculated for the bond strength data reported for different levels of factors: surface conditioning methods (control, physico-chemical, physical, chemical), cements (bis-GMA-, MDP- and 4-META-based resin cements, self-adhesive cements, glass ionomers), ageing with and without thermocycling (TC) and test methods (macro-shear, micro-shear, macro-tension, micro-tension). The final search provided 177 titles with abstracts. Additional abstract screening produced 72 articles, of which 54 were found to be potentially suitable for inclusion. After evaluation of the full text, 2 of them were eliminated. The selection process resulted in a final sample of 52 studies. In total, 169 different surface conditioning methods were investigated, mainly combinations of air abrasion protocols and adhesive promoters (primers or silanes). In total, the use of 5 types of cements and 4 test methods was reported. While 26 studies were carried out without thermocycling as aging, 26 of them employed thermocycling with several cycles. This review highlighted that the adhesion of luting cements is significantly influenced by the surface conditioning method ($p = 0.044$), type of cement ($p = 0.018$), test method ($p = 0.017$) and ageing condition ($p = 0.003$). In unconditioned control groups without thermocycling, the average bond strength values varied between 1.15 (IQR = 3.54) and 8.93 (IQR = 9), and 6.9 (IQR = 0) and 8.73 (IQR = 13.93) MPa for macroshear and macrotensil tests, respectively. After the physical conditioning method, the MDP monomer-based cement showed the highest bond values compared to other resin cements using the macrotensile (no TC: 34.2; IQR = 24.18 MPa, TC: 42.35; IQR = 0 MPa) or microtensile (no TC: 37.2; IQR = 41.5 MPa, TC: 17.1; IQR = 31.15 MPa) test method. Based on the results of this systematic review, it was concluded that greater adhesion can be expected after the physical-chemical conditioning of zirconium; resin cements based on MDP tend to show higher results than other types of cement when tested using macro- and micro-tensile tests. Zirconia adhesion studies and data reports require more standardization.

Satake et al. (2015) analyzed current scientific evidence on zirconium surface treatment methods, according to scientific literature from January 2007 to February 2012. Zirconium oxide frameworks have gained prominence among fixed prosthetic materials due to their physical, biological and aesthetic properties. However, the process of bonding this structure to dental cements is still a matter of debate. Zirconium oxide ceramics are characterized by having an extremely hard surface and no silica in their composition, making it impossible to use the standard treatment used for feldspathic ceramics. Various types of surface treatment have been investigated in an attempt to improve the cement/zirconia bond interface. The databases used were Medline, Pubmed, Web of Science and the Cochrane Library. After the bibliographic survey, 125,844 studies were found, of which only 376 were on the subject of the research; no clinical studies were found, only 'in vitro' studies. Inclusion and exclusion criteria were applied, leaving 21 articles for final analysis. After extracting the data, it was observed that the best results were found in the association of silica-coated sandblasting with metallic primers or silanes. It was not possible to carry out a quantitative analysis due to the heterogeneity of the studies in relation to the type of treatment, cement used, type of ageing, mechanical test, form of application of the thermocycling test, form of storage, among others. It is necessary to establish international standards for carrying out scientific research.

Bmicke et al. (2016) evaluated the bond strength of resin cements, after artificial aging by methods available in dental practice, for adhesive cementation to zirconium oxide ceramics. The specimens were standardized, consisting of composite resin cylinders (Rebilda SC, lot 1122213, VOCO; Cuxhaven, Germany) 3.3 mm in diameter which were bonded to pre-sintered zirconium oxide blocks (IPS e.max ZirCAD, Ivoclair Vivadent, Schan, Linchestein). The methods used to condition the zirconia surface were as follows: none (control); aluminium oxide blasting (50 µm, 10 mm, 10 sec, at 0.05; 0.10; 0.25 Mpa) (Alustral; Rodgan, Germany); tribochemical silica coating using the Rocatec system (3M-ESPE, Seefeld, Germany); silicatization using the Cojet system (3M-ESPE, Seefeld, Germany). The cementation systems were used in the following combinations: Panavia 21 + Clearfil Ceramic primer; Multilink Automix + Monobond Plus; BiFix QM + Ceramic Bond; ReliX Ultimate + Scotchbond Universal. After cementation, the specimens were stored in an incubator under 100% humidity at 37°C for 24 hours and subsequently divided into two subgroups. The samples in one subgroup were stored in distilled water at 37°C for 72 h, referred to as short-term ageing, before the tensile test. The other subgroup, referred to as the long-term ageing, was subjected to water storage at 37°C for 150 days in conjunction with thermocycling (Thermocycler TC 1, Willytec; Purgen, Germany) for 37,500 cycles (7500 cycles each after 25, 50, 75, 100, and 125 days) in distilled water at temperatures of 6.5°C and 60°C. The dwell time at each temperature was 45 seconds and the total transfer time was 7.5 seconds. The samples were then subjected to the tensile test, the data collected and analyzed by ANOVA analysis of variance. With the results obtained and the limitations of this study, it was concluded that: surface activation by the means mentioned in this study, with the use of coupling agents based on MDP and MPA associated with aluminum oxide blasting and silica blasting, with resin cements, improve the resin/zirconia bond strength. Adhesion is still a major challenge, as after ageing there was a significant reduction in the bond strength of the resin cement.

El-Ghany & Sherief (2016) carried out a study that aimed to look at aspects of the use of zirconium oxide in dentistry. Improved material strength, enhanced aesthetics, high biocompatibility give zirconium oxide a great possibility of being used for a wide range of promising clinical applications. This evaluation presents the different types of zirconium materials available for dental application, the effect of the machining processes with these materials, the aesthetics, cementation and application of the veneering ceramic in addition to the biological properties of these new materials. It was concluded that the use of zirconium oxide ceramics seems to be gaining a well-established place in today's clinical dentistry due to their exceptional physical and biological properties and the great improvement in CAD-CAM technology; a reliable choice of surface treatment and cement for cementing zirconium oxide contributes to the prevention of cracks. Resin cements are recommended because they have been shown to produce greater bond strength for both the zirconium and dentin surfaces when compared to conventional cements; because of the rapid development of both materials and processing technologies, the application of zirconium oxide-based prostheses can be seen as a promising alternative. However, dentists, researchers and dental technicians must work together to overcome the aesthetic limitations of zirconia materials.

Hallmann et al. (2016) in their study evaluated the effect of surface modifications on the tensile strength between zirconia ceramics and resin. The zirconium ceramic surfaces were treated with 150µm abrasive alumina particles, 150µm abrasive zirconia particles, argon-ion bombardment, gas plasma and piranha solution (H_2SO_4: H_2O_2 = 3: 1). The untreated surfaces were used as the control group. Tensile bond strength (TBS) values were measured after storage in water for 3 days and 150 days with an additional thermal cycling of 37,500 for artificial ageing. Statistical analyses were carried out using 1- and 3-criterion ANOVA, followed by comparison of means using the Tukey test. From the results obtained and evaluated, it was concluded that factors such as cleanliness, roughness and micromechanical interlock play an important role in the bond strength and long-term durability between a zirconia ceramic and a zirconia resin cement; the use of abrasive alumina particles has a positive effect on bond strength and durability due to increased cleanliness, roughness, micromechanical interlock and surface activity; the use of abrasive zirconium particles increased bond strength due to increased cleanliness and surface activity; the rough surface prepared by slip casting also had a positive effect on bond strength and long-term durability. In this case, TSB was the only factor that influenced bond strength and long-term durability. The use of abrasive zirconia particles instead of alumina particles and a surface prepared by slip casting shows promise as methods of reducing the defect of Y-TZP ceramic surfaces.

Luthra & Kaur (2016) reviewed the current literature on methods of bonding resin cement to ceramics with high flexural strength, such as zirconia-infiltrated alumina, densely sintered alumina and polycrystalline tetragonal zirconia ceramic partially stabilized with yttrium oxide (Y-TZP), with respect to strengthening cementation and bond durability. The keywords or phrases used were 'air particle abrasion', 'zirconia ceramic' and 'resin composite cements'. Studies from January 1989 to June 2015 were included. The literature showed that there are several techniques

available for surface treatments, but bond strength tests in different studies have produced conflicting results. Within the scope of this review, there is no evidence to support a universal ceramic surface treatment technique for adhesive cementation. A combination of chemical and mechanical treatments may be recommended. The use of tribochemical silica coating together with zirconia primers and cements containing phosphate monomers showed higher bond strength values. The hydrolytic stability of the resin ceramic bond should be improved.

Tzanakakis et al. (2016) conducted a systematic review, which aimed to classify and analyze existing methods and materials proposed to improve adhesion to zirconia surfaces. In the current literature, in vitro clinical studies examining the cement adhesion strength of zirconia ceramics from 1998 to 2014 were analyzed. A search was conducted using MEDLINE and PubMed, and a manual search was made for any relevant research papers from a dental school library. Studies evaluating only alumina restoration bonding or ceramic-zirconia bonding were excluded. A total of 134 publications were identified for analysis. Different adhesive techniques with different test methods were reviewed. The results were difficult to compare as the parameters varied in each research protocol. Based on the findings of this systematic review, the following conclusions were drawn: Aluminum oxide blasting (from 25 to 250 µm) is a reference method included in most research protocols; Tribochemical silica coating increases bonding capacity, especially when silanes are applied; adhesive monomers are necessary for chemical bonding; surface contamination and aging have negative effects on zirconium adhesion; the role of aging is important for most research protocols, but must be confirmed by clinical trials.

Zhao et al. (2016) states that creating a reliable and durable adhesion to the zirconia surface is difficult because it has limited use and that the introduction of functional monomers such as 10-methacryloyloxydecyl dihydrogen phosphate silane (MDP) appears to exert an improved bond strength to zirconia. The aim of this in vitro study was to evaluate the long-term adhesive strength of coupling systems and resin cement containing MDP for zirconia. To this end, the zirconia blocks were divided into 6 groups (n = 24) according to the 3 primers and cements to be bonded, as follows: Scotchbond Universal / RelyX Ultimate (SU / RU; consisting of primer containing MDP / cement without MDP); Clearfil ceramic primer / Panavia F (CCP / PAN; both consisting of MDP); and Z-Prime Plus / Duo-Link (ZP / DUO; containing MPA / without MDP), which were compared with 3 non-primer groups, RU, PAN and DUO. After bonding, each group was further divided into 3 subgroups (n = 8) according to the level of ageing: 24-hour storage in water at 37°C (24 hours); 30-day storage at 37°C. Followed by 3000 thermal cycles (30 days / TC). After ageing, they were subjected to shear strength testing and failure mode analysis was carried out. The data was analyzed using two-way ANOVA. After ageing, almost all primer/cement groups showed significantly higher adhesion strength than the related non-primed groups for each ageing level ($P < 0.05$), except for CCP/PAN versus PAN at 24h. SU/RU showed higher bond strength among the groups for all treatments ($P < 0.05$), except for CCP/PAN versus SU/RU at 30D/CT. Among the unselected groups, only RU was through 30 days / TC without premature detachment. At 24h and 30 days, the failure modes in SU/ RU and CCP/PAN were purely mixed, while the other groups were mainly adhesive, except RU. Based on this in vitro study, it was concluded that the presence of MDP in the cement was not significant in the long-term bond strength with zirconia; the SU/ RU primer/cement system had the highest initial and over time bond strength with zirconia; and slow thermal cycling tests are recommended to assess the longevity of low thermal conductivity materials such as zirconium oxide and composite resin.

Guilardi et al. (2017) aimed in this study to determine the effects of surface treatment with wear abrasion and low-temperature aging on the biaxial flexural strength, structural reliability, surface topography, roughness analysis and phase transformation of a polycrystalline tetragonal zirconia ceramic stabilized with itrium. Ceramic discs (15.0 × 1.2 ± 0.2 mm, VITA In-Ceram YZ) were prepared and randomly assigned to six groups according to two factors (n = 30): surface treatment by wear (Ctrl - no treatment, sintered powder; Xfine - wear with an extra-fine diamond drill - 30 µm; Coarse - wear with a coarse diamond drill - 151 µm) and "ageing" (without or with ageing: Ctrl LTD; Xfine LTD; Coarse LTD). Roughening was carried out in an oscillating motion with a contra-angle handpiece under constant cooling with water. The low temperature (LTD) was simulated in an autoclave at 134°C, under a pressure of 2 bar, for 20 hours. Roughness increased significantly after wear according to the size of the drill bit (Coarse > Xfine > Ctrl), and ageing had different effects (Ctrl = Ctrl LTD; Xfine > Xfine LTD; Coarse = Coarse LTD). Wear increased the monoclinic phase, and ageing led to an increase in the monoclinic phase in all groups. However, differences were observed in LTD. Weibull analysis showed a significant increase in characteristics after wear (Coarse = Xfine > Ctrl), while ageing had no deleterious impact. Neither wear nor ageing resulted in any deleterious impact on the reliability of the material. Thus, it was assessed that neither wear nor ageing led to a deleterious effect on the mechanical properties of Y-TZP ceramics, although a high monoclinic phase content and roughness were observed.

Pozzobon et al. (2017) investigated the effects of different surface conditioning methods on the strength of zirconia in biaxial bending, surface characteristics and fractographic analysis of a Y-TZP ceramic. The disk-shaped samples were fabricated and then randomly assigned to seven groups (n = 30). Control (CTRL): no treatment; tribochemical silica coating (TBS): specimens were blasted with silica-coated aluminum oxide particles (CoJet-Sand) for 10 s; silica nanofilm coating (SNF): specimens were coated with a 5 nm SiO2 nanofilm; and four low-fusion porcelain (GLZ) coating protocols: treatment with 10% fluoridic acid (HF) gel for 1 min (GLZ1), 5 min (GLZ5), 10 min (GLZ10) and 15 min (GLZ15). After the preparations and biaxial bending tests, the phase transformation, roughness, micro morphological changes, bending analysis tests and fractographic analyses were evaluated. X-ray diffraction (XRD) analysis showed that TBS promoted the highest monoclinic phase content. However, for the GLZ groups, XRD analysis was not sensitive enough to obtain an accurate reading of the phase transformation. The GLZ group showed the highest roughness values. The TBS group showed the highest strength characteristic, followed by SNF. These results suggest that the (TBS) and (SNF) treatments did not reduce mechanical properties, while (GLZ) led to a degradation in mechanical properties. They concluded that tribochemical treatment (TBS group) and silica nanofilm deposition (SNF group) did not degrade the mechanical properties of Y-TZP. Therefore, they can be recommended as a surface treatment for zirconium oxide. The application of low-fusion porcelain seems to promote deterioration in biaxial flexural strength. This deterioration may be due to factors such as the bi-layer that is formed, but it may also have been influenced by the method used.

3 PROPOSAL

The aim of this study was to evaluate the shear bond strength between two resin cements, RelyX U200 (3M ESPE) and Multilink (Ivoclair Vivadent), to titanium (Ti grade V alloy) and a zirconium oxide ceramic, both with treated and untreated surfaces.

The null hypothesis is that surface treatment by blasting with Aluminum Oxide associated with the use of Metal/Zirconia Primer does not influence the bond strength of the two cements tested on the surface of Titanium and Zirconium.

4 MATERIALS AND METHODS

This study received a Waiver of Submission to the Ethics Committee, issued by the Sao Leopoldo Mandic institution, whose protocol number is 2013/0159. This study used the ceramic system Zirconium Oxide stabilized with itrium oxide (Ceramil, Amann Girrbach, Curitiba, PR, Brazil) and Titanium Alloy grade V (Singular Dalton, Parnamirim, RN, Brazil). The systems used for cementation were "Multilink Sistem Pack" (Ivoclar Vivadent AG, FL-9494, Schann, Lichenstain) - Self-curing resin cement, "RelyX U200" (3M ESPE, Deutschland Gmbh/ D-82229 Seefeld, Germany) - Self-adhesive resin cement and silane coupling agent for metal and zirconia (Ivoclair - Vivadent) (Figure 1, 2, 3). A total of 80 samples (N = 80), forming the zirconia (N = 40) and titanium (N = 40) groups. The groups were subdivided into eight subgroups (n = 10) as shown in Table 1:

Table 1: Classification of groups.

Group	Material	CEMENT	SURFACE TREATMENT
1	Zirconia	U200	YES
2	Zirconia	U200	NO
3	Zirconia	MULTILINK	YES
4	Zirconia	MULTILINK	NO
5	Titanium	U200	YES
6	Titanium	U200	NO
7	Titanium	MULTILINK	YES
8	Titanium	MULTILINK	NO

Source: Own authorship.

The materials used in this work with their respective descriptions such as trade name, manufacturer, characteristics, chemical composition and batch number are shown in Table 2.

Table 2 - Materials used in this work.

	Manufacturer	***Features***	***Composition***	***Lot***
Multilink	Ivoclar Vivadent	Resin cement self-curing chemical	*Organic matrix of* ethoxylated Bis-EMA, UDMA, BIS-GMA, HEMA.	805946
Metal/Zirconia	Ivoclar Vivadent	polymerization	*Inorganic particles* of barium glass, tri-.	R60214

		Primer for metals and	ytterbium fluoride, mixed spheroidal oxides. Sizes from 0.25 - 3.0 mm (average 0.9 mm) and total volume of inorganic particles of 39,7%.	
Primer		Zirconia	Phosphonic acid acrylate and agents cross-linked methacrylates in a organic solution	
RelyX U200	3M ESPE	Resin cement polymer self-adhesive - dual-layering	*Base paste:* silane-treated glass powder, 2-propenoic acid, 2-methyl 1, 1'-[1-(hydroxy-methyl)-1, 2-ethanodly] ester, dimethacrylate with silane, glass fiber, sodium persulate and t-butyl per-3, 5, 5-trimethylhexanoate. *Catalyst paste:* silane-treated glass powder, substituted dmethacrylate, silane-treated silica, sodium p-toluenesulphate, 1-benzyl-5-phenyl-basic acid, calcium salts, 1, 12-dodecane dimethacrylate, hydroxide, sodium p-toluenesulphate, sodium p-toluenesulphate, sodium p-toluenesulphate, sodium p-toluenesulphate, sodium p-toluenesulphate, sodium p-toluenesulphate.	1329500659
Zirconium oxide	*Ceramill*	*Zirconia Oxide Polycrystals Stabilized with Itria*		392508
Titanium alloy	*Singular Dalton*	*TI-6Al-4V (grade v)*		*700356S*

Source: Own authorship.

Figura 1 - Multilink self-curing resin cement (Ivoclar - Vivadent).

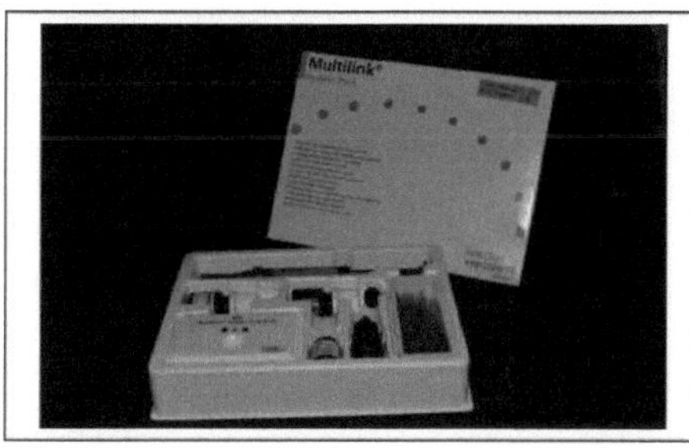

Source: Own authorship.

Figura 2 - RelyX U200 self-adhesive resin cement.

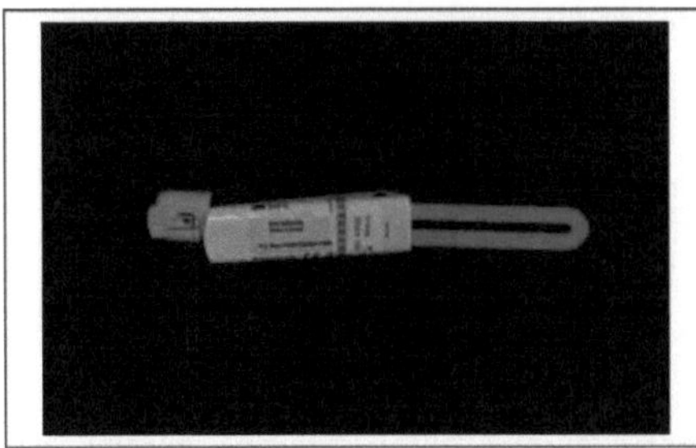

Source: Own authorship.

Figura 3 - Silane coupling agent for metal and zirconia (Ivoclar - Vivadent).

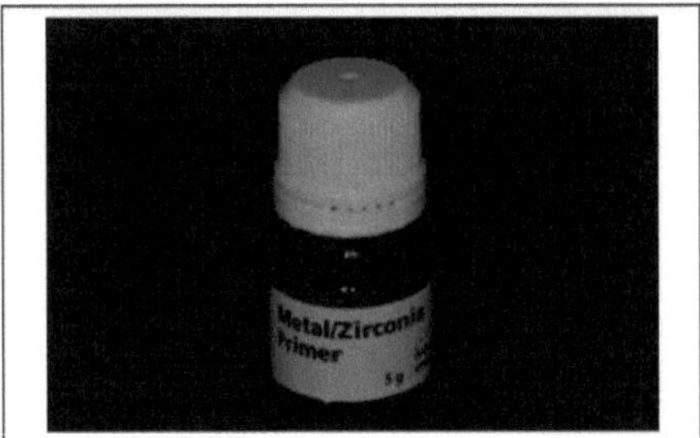

Source: Own authorship.

4.1 Obtaining the specimens

4.1.1 Obtaining zirconia oxide samples

A block of zirconium oxide stabilized by itrium was purchased pre-sintered, with a diameter of 100.0 mm and a thickness of 8.0 mm (Ceramill, Amann Girrbach, Curitiba, Brazil), which was cut and machined to obtain 20 square tablets measuring 7.0 x 7.0 x 8.0 mm. These tablets were cut in half and sent to the Zirkonzahn sintering furnace (Zirkonzahn, Gais, Italy) for 8 hours at a temperature of 1500°C. They were then cooled at room temperature, resulting in 40 pellets measuring approximately 7.0 x 7.0 x 3.0 mm. There was a reduction in the volume of the tablets due to the structural physical contraction of the Zirconium in the sintering process. The tablets were made by Laboratório Padilha (Vitória, Brazil) (figure 4).

4.1.2 Obtaining the titanium samples

40 grade V titanium alloy cylindrical inserts were purchased measuring 5.5 mm in diameter by 3.0 mm thick, prepared and machined by the manufacturer (Singular Dalton, Pamamirim-RN, Brazil) (figure 4).

Figure 4 - Titanium and Zirconium specimens.

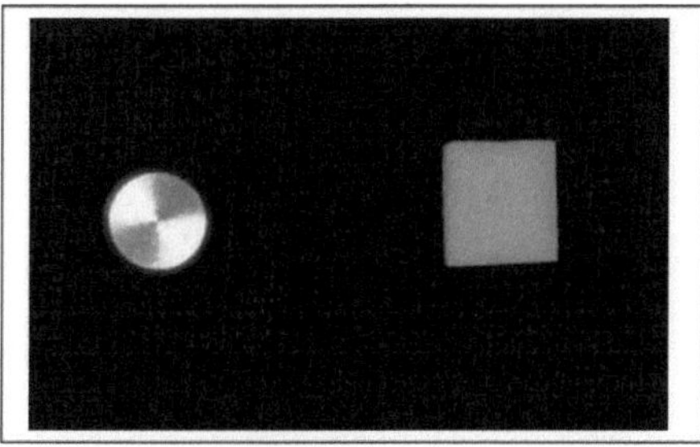

Source: Own authorship.

4.1.3 Inclusion

All the zirconium oxide and titanium alloy inserts were embedded in VipiFlash colorless self-curing acrylic resin (VIPI Indùstria e Comércio, Pirassununga - Sao Paulo - Brazil) (Figure 5) inside a PVC tube ½ inch in diameter and 30 mm high. To do this, a glass plate was used, on which two markings were made: one along the diameter of the PVC tube and the other centered with an overhead projector pen. The ceramic inserts and PVC tubes were glued to the surface of the glass plate at the appropriate markings, using Prit glue stick (Henkel Chile S.A. Santiago, Chile) (Figure 6 a, b, c). The acrylic resin was handled according to the manufacturer's specifications and poured to the brim inside the PVC tubes, over the zirconium oxide and titanium alloy inserts (Fig. 7 a, b, c).

Figura 5 - Self-curing resin for specimen inclusion.

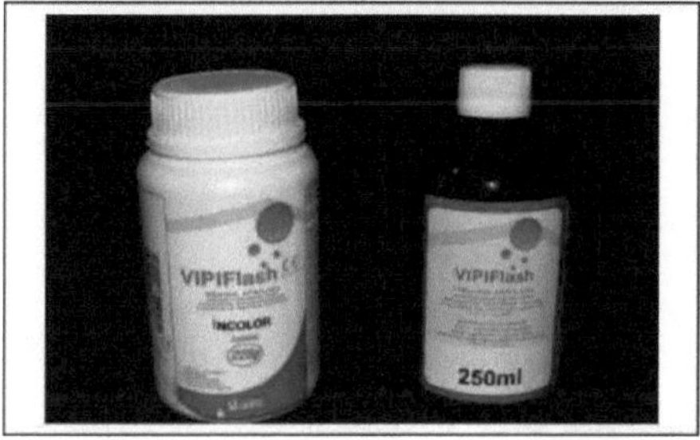

Source: Own authorship.

Figura 6 - Demarcation of samples.

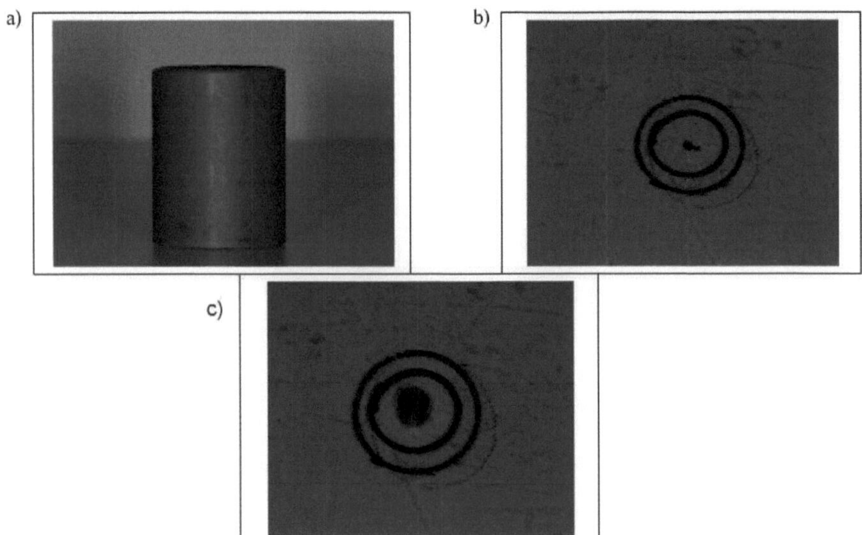

Legend: a) PVC tube; b) Demarcations on glass plate; c) Titanium sample positioned to be included in the resin.

Source: Own authorship.

Figure 7 - Inclusion of samples.

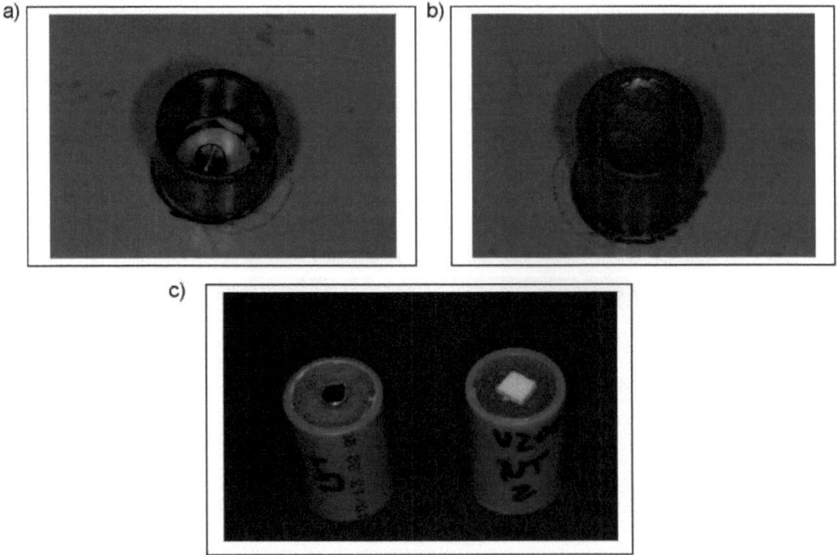

Caption: a) Titanium sample and tube positioned for inclusion; b) Resin inclusion

c) Titanium and Zirconia specimens.

Source: Own authorship.

1.1.4 Obtaining the Silicone Condensation Matrix

The silicone matrix is necessary to obtain standardized samples of the resin cements on the titanium and zirconia surfaces. A metal matrix measuring 11.0 mm in diameter by 3 mm in height was used to make the silicone matrix. It was fitted over the PVC tube, delimiting the area needed to make the silicone matrix. A second matrix, with a central perforation of 3 mm in diameter, was used as a perforation guide for the silicone matrix (Figure 8 a, b, c). A portion of Zetalabor (Zhermark Techinacal, Badia Polesine, Italy) condensation silicone base paste/catalyst paste (Figure 9) was dispensed and manipulated according to the manufacturer's recommendations, and inserted inside the first metal matrix. After it had completely set, the second matrix was attached to the top of the first matrix, where a perforation was made in the central region with a 3.0 mm diameter Bosch drill (Bosch AS, Lisbon, Portugal), delimiting the area/volume of the inserted cement (Figures 10 and 11).

Figure 8 - Matrix assembly:

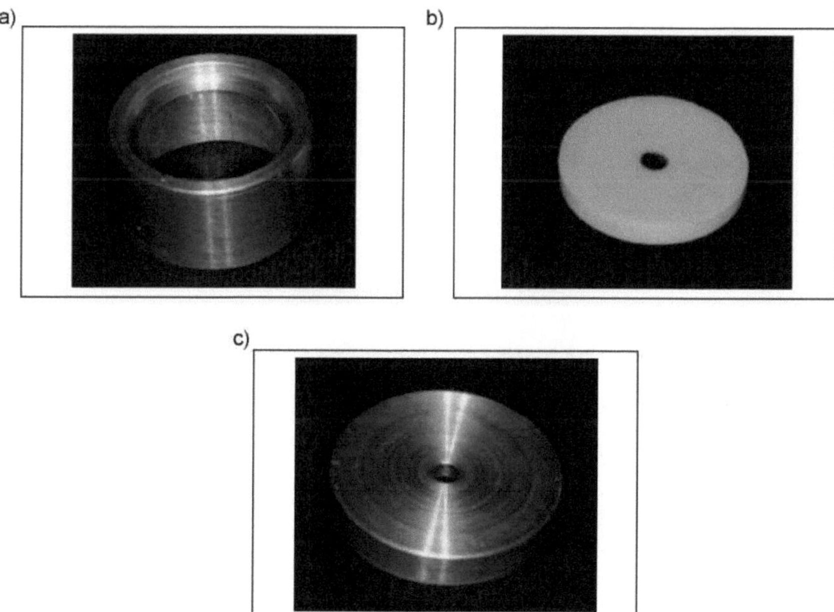

Legend: a) Positioning ring on the PVC tube; b) Silicone matrix for inserting the cement; c) Guide matrix for drilling the silicone matrix.

Source: Own authorship.

Figure 9 - laboratory silicone for the matrix.

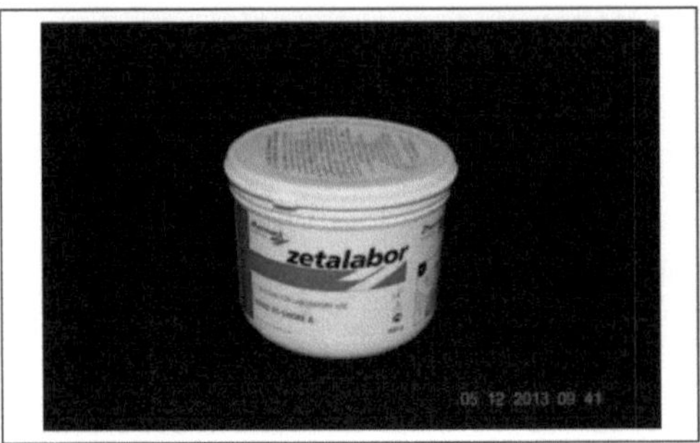

Source: Own authorship.

Figure 10 - Making the metal matrix for inserting the cement.

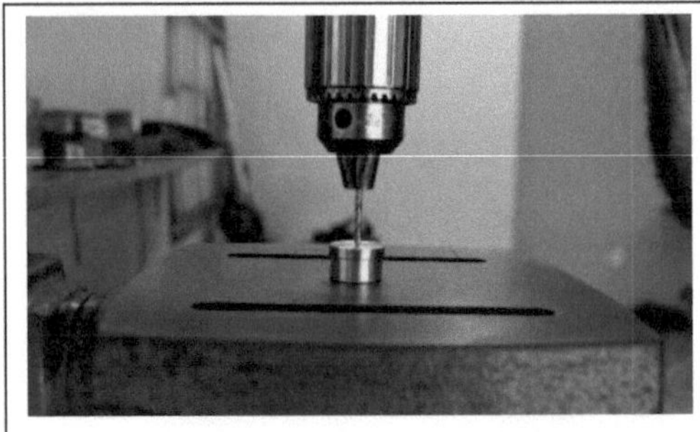

Source: Own authorship.

Figure 11 - Sequence of matrix assembly.

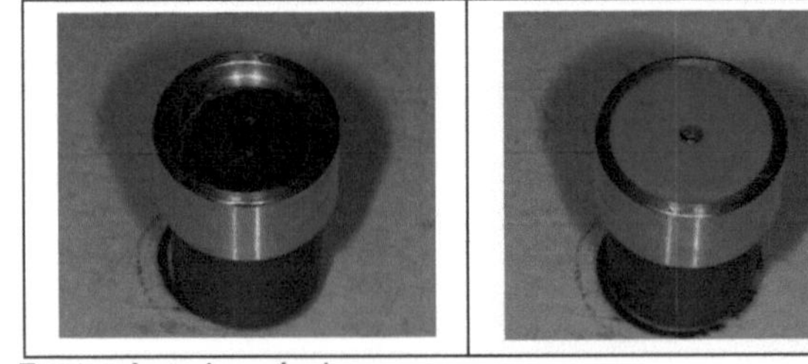
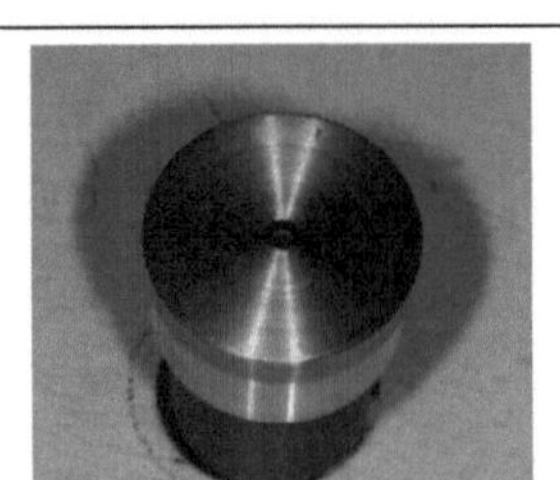

Source: Own authorship.

4.1.5 Surface treatment

The titanium specimens were taken to the polishing machine (Arotec Ind. e Comércio,

Aropol 2V, Sâo Paulo, Brazil), where they were smoothed and polished using Wertordry (3M ESPE) 320, 400, 600, 800 and 1200 grit sandpaper in sequence, for about 30 seconds each, at a speed of 600 rpm (Figure 12). Forty titanium and zirconium specimens received no surface treatment and the remaining forty specimens received surface treatment in accordance with previous studies: aluminum oxide blasting with 50µm granules, at 0.25 Mpa pressure, 10.0 mm apart for 10 seconds (Figures 13 and 14). All the samples were washed with an air/water jet for 30 seconds, then bathed for 10 minutes in distilled water in an ultrasonic cleaner (Cristófoli, Campo Mourâo, Paranà, Brazil) and then dried with an air jet free of water and oil (Figure 15).

Figura 12 - Polisher.

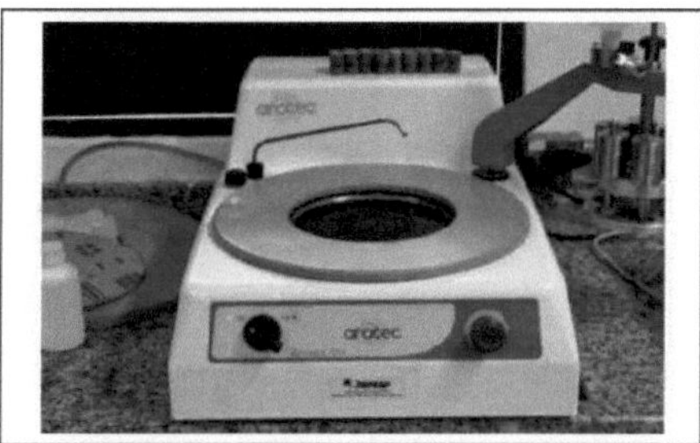

Source: Own authorship.

Figura 13 - Aluminum oxide blasting machine.

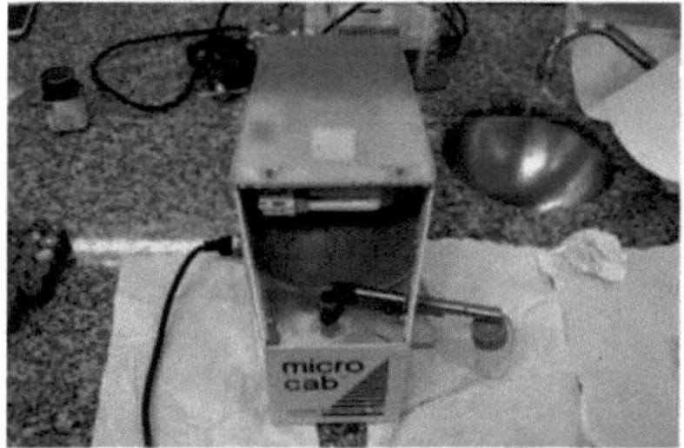

Source: Own authorship.

Figura 14 - Sandblasted specimens.

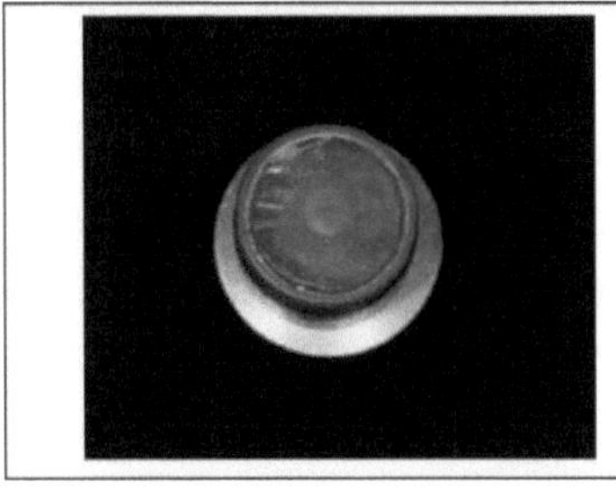

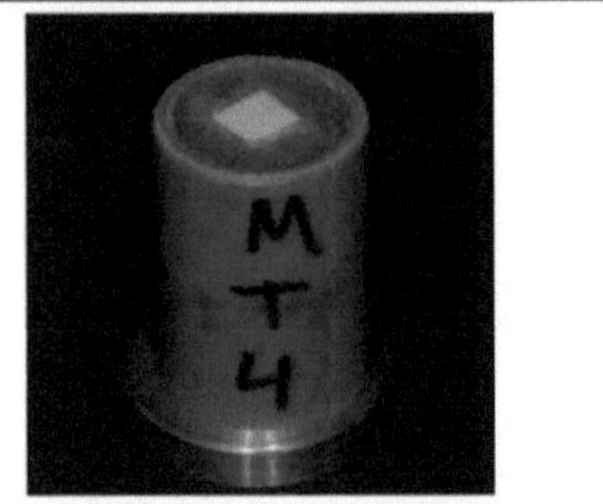

Source: Own authorship.

Figura 15 - Ultrasonic cleaner for cleaning the specimens.

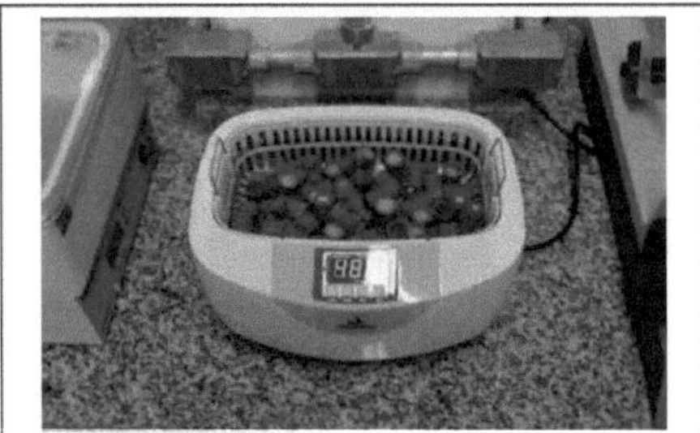

Source: Own authorship.

4.1.6 Application of Metal/Zirconia Primer

Using a hand-held applicator supplied by the manufacturer, a drop of the Metal/Zirconia Primer was dispensed onto the surface of the Titanium and Zirconium, forming a thin layer and left to react for 180 seconds, the time recommended by the manufacturer. It was then dried with water- and oil-free air. This material was only used with Multilink cement, as RelyX U200 cement is not necessary because it is self-conditioning and self-adhesive.

4.1.7 Cementing

Once the surface treatment had been completed, the first metal matrix associated with the silicone matrix was individually fitted into the PVC tube to delimit the area where the resin cement would adhere to the zirconia oxide and titanium alloy tablets. With the matrices in place, the pastes were dispensed from the double-pressure syringes onto the manipulation block and mixed in a 1:1 ratio, according to the manufacturer's instructions. The two portions of resin cement were manipulated with a plastic spatula for 20 seconds and the excess was inserted with a composite resin spatula (Duflex- SSWite) (Figure 16). A strip of polyester was cut to fit the surface of the matrix, with the aim of regularizing the surface of the cement and preventing contact with oxygen. To stabilize this matrix, the second matrix was placed on top of it, acting as a standardized weight for all the samples to be cemented and then left for 6 minutes to set (figures 17 and 18). They were then photoactivated for 40 seconds with a light-curing device (Ultra lux - Dabi

Atlanta), only for inserts with RelyX U200 cement, as Multilink cement is self-curing. The cementing protocols were based on the guidelines of their respective manufacturers, and the handling, working and initial setting times were the same. The matrix was then removed from the specimens (figure 19).

Figura 16 - Material for handling resin cement.

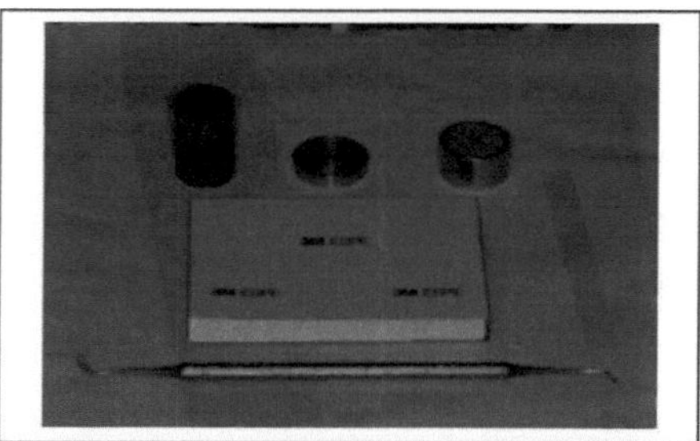

Source: Own authorship.

Figura 17 - Cement inserted into the matrix and polyester matrix positioned over the cement.

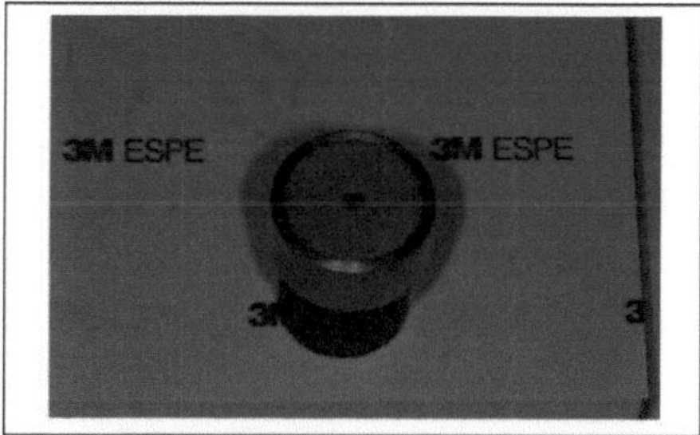

Source: Own authorship.

Figura 18 - The second matrix as a weight on the matrix, providing the same standard conditions.

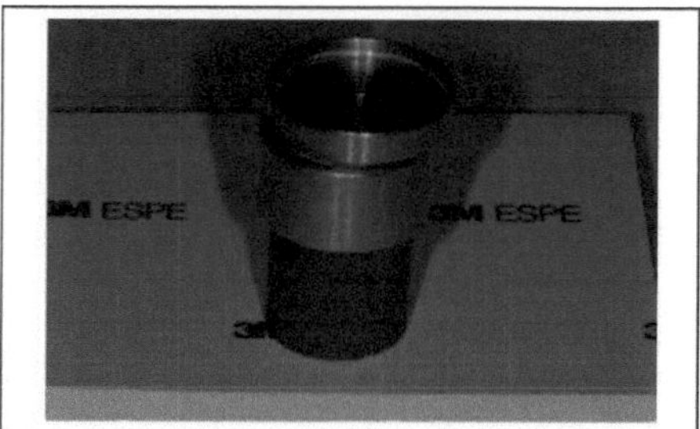

Source: Own authorship.

Figura 19 - Cement polymerized without matrix.

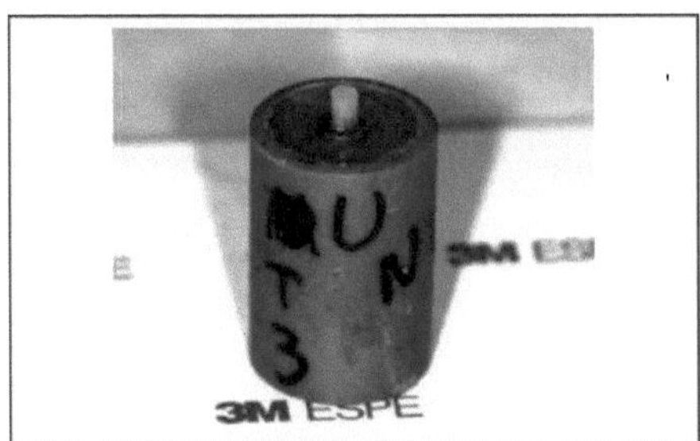

Source: Own authorship.

4.1.8 Thermocycling

A thermal cycling simulation machine (MSCT, Sâo Carlos, Brazil) was used to carry out the thermocycling (Figure 20). To avoid losses during the process, the specimens were placed and contained in a tulle bag. The samples were stored for 24 hours in distilled water at 37°C. Then, 1,000 thermal cycles of artificial ageing were carried out, varying from 5°C to 55°C, each bath lasting 30 seconds, with a time of 5 seconds from one bath to the next. The samples were again stored for 24 hours in distilled water at 37°C (Figure 21).

Figura 20 - Thermocycling device.

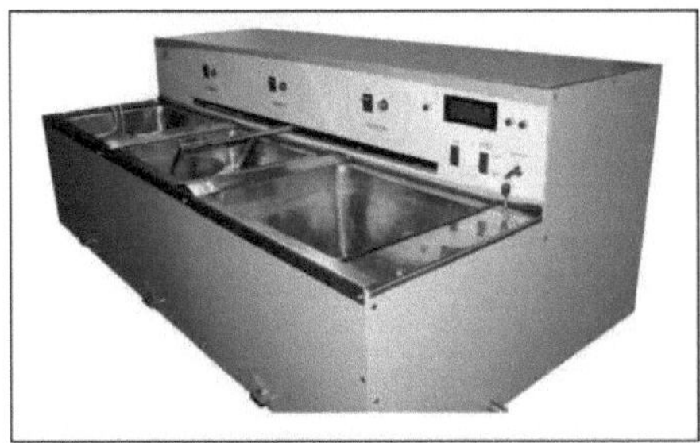

Source: Manufacturer.

Figura 21 - Specimen after thermocycling.

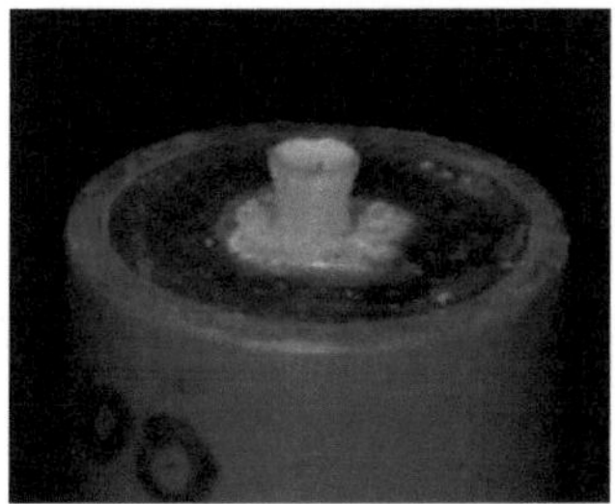

Source: Own authorship.

4.2 Shear bond strengths

4.2.1 Mechanical test

The mechanical shear test was carried out using an EMIC universal testing machine model DL 2000 (Sâo José dos Pinhais-Pr), with a load cell of 1961.33 N, with a mono angled chisel at a speed of 0.5 mm/min and with values recorded in Mpa (figure 22). The specimens were fixed to the machine so that the cylinders remained perpendicular to the action of the force applied by the chisel at the ceramic-resin cement adhesive interface (Figure 23 a, b, c).

The machine is connected to a computer and the test was monitored using software (TESC version 3.1, Instron Brasil, Sâo José dos Espinhais, Brazil) for test treatments. The monitor shows the relationship between the applied load and the displacement at the moment of fracture and is represented graphically. At the moment of fracture, the movement stops and the data is processed for analysis.

Figura 22 - EMIC universal testing machine.

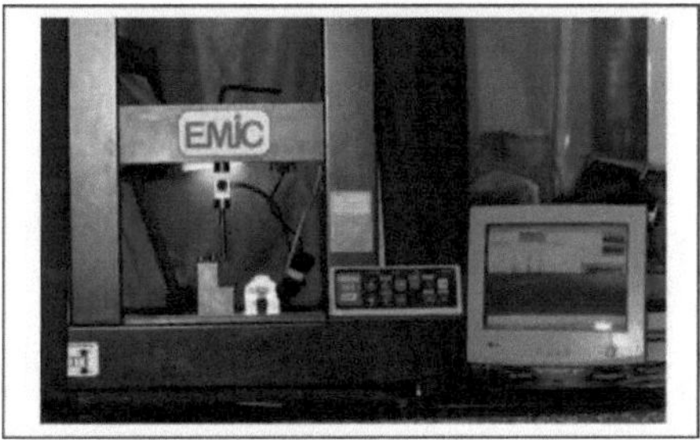

Source: Own authorship.

Figura 23 - Mechanical shear test.

a) b) c)

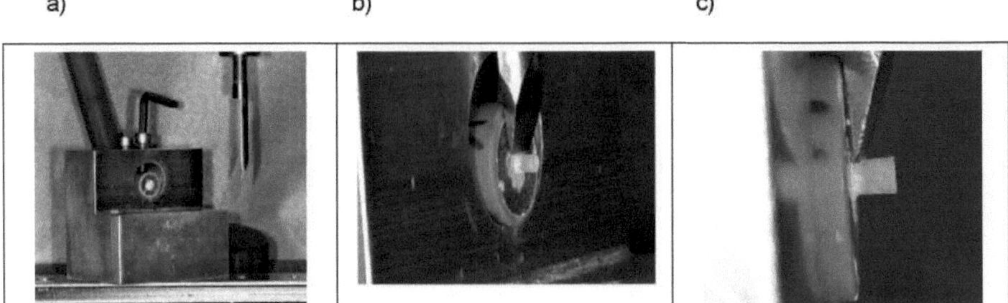

Caption: a) specimen positioned; b) blade positioned; c) moment of test.

4.2.2 Checking fault types

The types of flaws in the specimens were identified using a 40x magnification stereoscopic magnifier (Tec Nival). The images were classified as shown in Table 1.

Table 1: Classification of failure modes.

Groups	Adhesive	cement cohesive	Mixed
Zr/U200/Treated	x		
Zr/U200/Not Treated	x		
Zr/Multilink/Treated	x		
Zr/Multilink/Not Treated	x		
Ti/U200/Treated	x	X	
Ti/U200/Not Treated	x	X	x
Ti/Multilink/Treated	x		x
Ti/Multilink/Not Treated			x

4.2.3 Statistical Analysis

The bond strength values were subjected to three-way analysis of variance. Tukey's test was applied for multiple comparisons. The failure modes observed in the samples were analyzed descriptively. SPSS 20 (SPSS Inc., Chicago, IL, USA) was used for the statistical calculations, with a significance level of 5%.

5 RESULTS

Table 2 shows the descriptive analysis, in terms of means and standard deviations, of the shear bond strength values obtained using zirconium oxide ceramic stabilized with itrium oxide and grade V titanium, according to whether or not surface treatment and resin cement had been carried out. Five specimens were lost during the thermocycling process, one zirconium and four titanium.

Table 2 - Means and standard deviations of bond strength values according to material, surface treatment and resin cement.

Material	Surface	Resin cement	N	Joint strength (Mpa)
Ceramics of Zirconium oxide	Treated	RelyX U200	10	4,25 (1,00)
		Multilink	10	4,45 (2,17)
	Untreated	RelyX U200	10	4,98 (1,18)
		Multilink	9	3,43 (2,80)
Titanium	Treated	RelyX U200	10	17,86 (3,86)
		Multilink	9	16,11 (10,08)
	Untreated	RelyX U200	8	2,35 (0,71)
		Multilink	9	4,35 (2,64)

Source: Author

The three-way analysis of variance revealed that there was no significant three-way interaction between the variables *Material*, *Surface treatment* and *Resin cement* ($p = 0.066$). The two-way interaction *Material* x *Surface* proved to be significant ($p < 0.001$). The Tukey test used to dismantle this interaction showed that there was no significant difference between zirconium oxide ceramic and titanium in terms of bond strength when surface treatment was removed, regardless of the resin cement used (table 3 and graph 1). On the other hand, when surface treatment was carried out, titanium provided significantly higher bond strength values than zirconium oxide ceramic. Tukey's test also showed that zirconium oxide ceramics did not show any increase in bond strength after surface treatment, regardless of the resin cement used (table 3 and graph 1). In contrast, for titanium, surface treatment significantly increased its bond strength.

Table 3 - Means and standard deviations of bond strength values according to material and surface treatment, regardless of resin cement.

Material	Surface	
	Treated	Untreated
Zirconium oxide ceramics	4.35 (1.65) **Ba**	4.04 (2.34) **Aa**
Titanium	16.18 (8.07) **Aa**	2.82 (2.32) **Ab**

Caption: Distinct upper case letters indicate a significant difference between materials within each column. Distinct lowercase letters indicate a significant difference between treated and untreated surfaces within each row.

Source: Author

Graph 1 - Column diagram of average bond strength values according to material, surface treatment and resin cement (vertical bars indicate standard deviations).

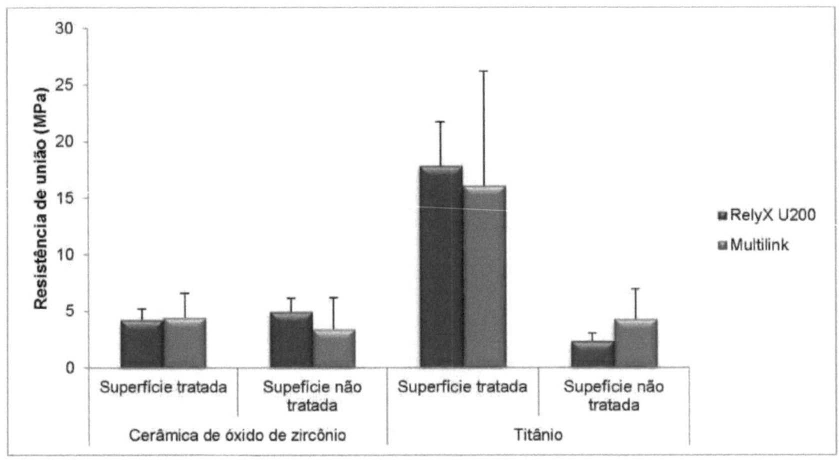

Source: Author

The three-way analysis of variance also indicated that there was no significant two-way interaction between the variables *Material* and Resin *cement* (p = 0.935), as well as between the variables *Surface treatment* and *Resin cement* (p = 0.418). There was also no significant difference in the bond strength values provided by RelyX U200 and Multilink resin cements (p = 0.444), regardless of whether treated or untreated zirconium oxide ceramic or titanium was used.

As for the failure mode, as shown in graph 2, when zirconium oxide ceramic was used, the ruptures were exclusively adhesive, regardless of whether or not the surface of this material had been treated and regardless of the cementing agent. For titanium, adhesive failures accounted for 60 to 90% of the rupture modes in the groups in which the surface was treated (regardless of the resin cement) and in the group in which surface treatment was omitted and RelyX U200 cement was used. Cohesive ruptures were only observed in the group in which the titanium was treated and cemented with Multilink, which had 20% of samples with cohesive fracture of the cement. Exclusively mixed failures were observed in the group in which the titanium was untreated and cemented with Multilink.

Graph 2 - Column diagram of failure modes by material, surface treatment and resin cement.

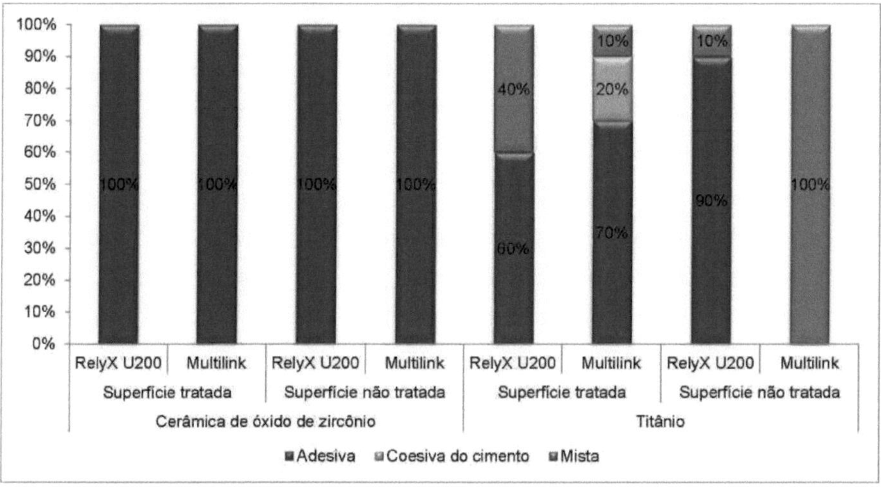

Source: Author

6 DISCUSSION

The success of cementing a ceramic crown on natural teeth is determined by the strength and durability of the bond formed between the tooth surface, the cementing agent and the ceramic used. Due to the wide variety of adhesive systems, resin cements and the different methods used to evaluate these materials, there is no consensus in the literature as to which would be the best combination that would lead to a more durable bond strength, the specific material to be cemented and the adhesive cement system to be used must be considered (Thompson et al., 2011; Belo et al., 2013; Mosele, Borba, 2014; Papia et al., 2014; Souza et al., 2014; Ozcan, Bernasconi, 2015; Satake et al., 2015; Luthra, Kaur, 2016, Tzanakakis et al., 2016).

The surface treatment of a material aims to clean and prepare the surface, creating microretentions where the material to be used on its surface will be favored by the mechanical engagement between the substrate and the cement. Micromechanical retention is determined by the topography of the surface to be cemented to the zirconium oxide restoration. Depending on the technique used, the roughness of the surface can vary, as a rougher surface will affect the wettability of the bonding agents to the material, allowing the cement to flow in the microretentions, favoring the quality of the mechanical bond between the cement and the zirconium (Mirmohammadi et al., 2010; Shahim, Kern, 2010; Mosele, Borba, 2014; Amaral et al., 2014; Inokoshi et al., 2014; Papia et al., 2014; Ozcan, Vallittu, 2003; Ozcan, Bernasconi, 2015; Satake et al., 2015; Hallmann et al., 2016; Tzanakakis et al., 2016; Pozzobon et al. 2017).

The mechanical surface treatment used in this study was Aluminum Oxide blasting with particle sizes of 50µm, pressure of 0.25 Mpa, exposure time of 10 sec. at a distance of 10 mm. This method requires a simpler technique and equipment that is easy to use. When the surface treatment was carried out, titanium provided more significant strength values and when this treatment was carried out on zirconium, there was no increase in bond strength. This was proven by the failure modes for zirconium oxide, which were 100% adhesive, regardless of the cement used and whether or not the surface treatment was carried out. This treatment showed no statistically significant difference for the zirconium surface, in contrast to the study by Shahim and Kern (2010) which, using the same surface treatment, promoted an increase in bond strength. Factors such as the exposure time of the surface to be blasted were what differentiated the two studies, as a time of 15 seconds was used with the same particle size, pressure and distance. Yang et al. (2010) achieved good results with the same blasting methodology as this study, but used a primer containing MDP, which according to Wolfart et al. (2007) and Gomes et al. (2013), provides better results regardless of the type of blasting and particle size. Qeblawi et al. (2010) stated that aluminum oxide blasting associated with primer containing MDP are promising, and that MDP (10-methacryloxydecyl dihydrogen phosphate) only has a durable bond when it is preceded by a surface treatment that provides mechanical retention, confirmed by Yang et al. (2010). According to a study by Yun et al. (2010) and Inokoshi et al. (2014), the use of cements and metallic primer alone is not sufficient for a lasting bond with zirconium cementation, and it is necessary to sandblast the surface in order to improve the levels of mechanical engagement.

Almeida et al. (2010) compared the blasting of aluminum oxide with particle sizes of 30, 50 and 110µm, with the 30 and 110µm particles coated with silica. The treatment with 110µm particles obtained the best results for the titanium surface. In the work by Taira et al. (1998), the surface treatment of titanium with an aluminium oxide jet had adequate strength and durability, but it has been shown that an excess layer of oxides can interfere with the durability of cementation. Future studies are suggested to evaluate the effects of blasting with larger particles on the surface of zirconia ceramics, as according to Luthardt et al. (2003), microcracks and flaws in the surface are induced by machining and handling, which can generate stress concentrators with possible future unforeseen events, with the association of the method for promoting mechanical retention, as confirmed by the studies by Mosel and Borba (2014) and Tzanakakis et al. (2016).

Studies have concluded that not only prior cleaning, roughening and surface activation, but also adhesive bonding and the use of resin composites containing MDP (10-methacryloxydecyl dihydrogen phosphate) are necessary for a durable bond to densely sintered zirconium oxide ceramics (Wolfart et al. 2007; Belo et al., 2013; Mosele, Borba, 2014; Souza et al, 2014; Ahn et al, 2015; Ozcan, Bernasconi, 2015; Hallmann et al, 2016; Zhao L et al, 2016). Studies that used a combination of mechanical and chemical methods showed higher bond strength values than studies that used these methods alone (Luthra, Kaur, 2016). The studies by Aboushelib et al. (2009) and Tzanakakis et al. (2016) concluded that the stability of the resin/zirconia bond is directly related to the chemistry of the materials used, including the initiators. Regarding chemical retention, different cementation systems have been proposed for bonding zirconium oxide ceramics in an attempt to achieve reliable adhesion. Under appropriate conditions, resin cements provide a stronger bond with better physical properties than conventional cements (Amarai et al., 2014; Mosel, Borba, 2014; Inokoshi et al., 2014; Papia et al., 2014; Ozcan, Vallittu, 2003;

Ozcan, Bernasconi, 2015; Luthra, Kaur, 2016; Hallmann et al., 2016; Tzanakakis et al., 2016; Pozzobon et al. 2017). Coupling agents promote the bonding of the cement to the substrate where, in addition to promoting surface wettability, they bond the substrate to the cement through their bifunctional molecules (Schneider et al., 2007). In general, silanes increase the wettability of an inorganic surface, allowing better cement flow through the surface and seem to improve micromechanical retention with low-viscosity resin cements (Tzanakakis et al., 2016). Surface conditioning and silanization are a standard laboratory protocol for dental restorations and their repair (Lung & Matinlinna, 2012).

Primers based on MPA (Phosphoric Acid Monomer) have multifunctional phosphoric acid methacrylates in their organic matrix, or simply acid monomers that interact with the hydroxyapatite of dental structures and should interact with zirconium. However, there are no reports in the literature that explain in detail how this interaction could occur. Phosphorylated methacrylates have a pH below 2 and, as with self-etching adhesives, when they come into contact with water or tooth moisture, they react with hydroxyapatite, increasing bond strength values (Oyague et al., 2009; Behr et al., 2011; Attia & Kern, 2011; Lung & Matinlinna, 2012; Amaral et al., 2014). The silane agent used in this study was Metal/Zirconia Primer (Ivoclair-

Vivadent) based on MPA, supplied by the Multilink cement kit, where the samples separated for the use of Multilink cement received this silanization treatment. Studies by Piascik et al. (2009), Aboushelib et al. (2009), Attia, Kern (2011), Amaral et al. (2014), Bomicke et al. (2016), standardized their silanizations with the MPA-based coupling agent used. One problem with the clinical use of zirconia components is the difficulty of achieving adequate adhesion to synthetic substrates or natural tissues (Thompsom et al., 2011; Bomicke et al., 2016). Therefore, no bonding concept can offer strong and reliable long-term bonding between resin and zirconia, which can withstand oral loading conditions (Behr et al., 2011).

For the zirconium samples in this study, surface treatment did not lead to significant values, as the values did not increase after surface treatment and remained low, regardless of the resin cement used. Piascik et al. (2009) state that not only surface treatment but also the addition of coupling initiating agents is necessary in order to achieve a stronger and longer-lasting bond between the substrate and the cement. This was proven by Matinlinna et al. (2006 abc.) in their studies, which tested and proved other coupling agents associated with other surface treatment techniques. As for titanium, the surface treatment influenced the result by significantly increasing the bond strength values, regardless of the cement used. This was proven by the failure modes, which were adhesive, cohesive and mixed, with cohesive failures occurring only with Multilink cement associated with the surface treatment.

MDP-based resin cements tend to show higher results than other types of cements when tested. Since the current results are controversial, the use of phosphonic-acid-base silane primers and MDP-based cements or self-adhesive cements that react directly with the oxides present on the zirconium surface are considered good alternatives to associate with air-abrasion systems (Ozcan, Bernasconi, 2015). This study used two different cement systems: the self-curing Multilink (Ivoclair/Vivadent) and the self-adhesive RelyX U200 (3M-ESPE) with dual polymerization. Because they were self-adhesive, the samples to be cemented with RelyXU200 cement were not silanized. For both materials used in this study, the results did not depend on the resin cement. Kim et al. (2011) made comparisons between various resin cements and concluded that surface energy parameters should be considered when evaluating cement adhesive properties with zirconia ceramics. Aleisa et al. (2013) confirmed that cementation was not influenced by the different types of resin cements. Mirmohammadi et al. (2010) were unable to detect any statistical difference between the resin cements using the shear test.

The aging test is an important factor that must be taken into account when developing research, as it negatively influences the zirconium/cement interface due to the hydrolytic degradation suffered by both parts (Satake et al., 2015). Among the mechanical testing methods used to assess bond strength, the most widely used in the literature are shear, micro-shear, tensile and micro-tensile tests (Inokoshi et al., 2014). Another very controversial issue is the selection of the mechanical test, as the results of microtensile and shear tests cannot be transferred to clinical situations, but they can compare and classify bonding concepts applied under identical conditions (Behr et al., 2011). Shear tests are more widely used than other tests, but there is a wide variation in the results obtained using similar tests and materials in different laboratories (Qeblawi et al., 2010; Yun et al., 2010; Behr et al., 2011; Matinlinna et al., 2011; Kawai et al., 2012; Tzanakakis et al., 2016). This study used the shear test, which is not only the most widely used test, but also the one best suited to comparing the different conditions evaluated.

7 CONCLUSION

Based on the methodology applied and the results obtained from this study, it was concluded that:

1. Surface treatment with aluminum oxide blasting was effective for titanium, increasing the bond strength values of Multilink and RelyX U200 cements. With zirconium, surface treatment did not alter the bond strength values of Multilink and RelyX U200 cements.

2. Both cements were sufficient to increase the cement bond strength values on the titanium surface. The opposite occurred on the zirconium surface, where the cements were not sufficient to increase the cement bond strength values,

3. The null hypothesis was confirmed for zirconia and denied for titanium.

8 REFERENCES[I]

Aboushelib MN, Mirmohamadi H, Matinlinna JP, Kukk E, Ounsi HF, Salamehf Z. Innovations in bonding to zirconia-based materials. Part II: Focusing on chemical interactions. Dental Materials.2009; 25: 989 - 993.

Ahn JS, Yi YA, Lee Y, Seo DG. Shear Bond Strength of MDP-Containing SelfAdhesive Resin Cement and Y-TZP Ceramics: Effect of Phosphate MonomerContaining Primers. BioMed Research International. 2015. Article ID 389234. 6 pages.

Aleisa K, Alwazzan K, Al-Dwairi ZN, Almoharib H, Alshabib A, Aleid A, Lynch E. Retention of zirconium oxide copings using different types of luting agents. Journal of Dental Sciences. 2013; xx, 1-7.

Almeida AAJ, Fonseca RG, Haneda IG, Abi-Rached FO, Adabo GL. Effect of Surface Treatments on the Bond Strength of a Resin Cement to Commercially Pure Titanium. Braz Dent J. 2010; 21(2): 111-116.

Amaral M, Belli R, Cesar PF, Valandro LF, Petschelt A, Lohbauerm U. The potential of novel primers and universal adhesives to bond to zirconia. Journal of Dentistry. 2014. 42: 90 - 98.

Attia A, Kern M. Long-term resin bonding to zirconia ceramic with a new universal primer. J Prosthet Dent. 2011; 106:319-327.

Behr M, Proff P, Kolbeck C, Langrieger S, Kunze J, Handel G, Rosentritt M. The bond strength of the resin-to-zirconia interface using different bonding concepts. Journal of the Mechanical Behavior of Biomedical Materials. 2011; 4: 2-8.

Belo YD, Sonza QN, Borba M, Bona AD. Ytria-stabilized tetragonal zirconia: mechanical behavior, adhesion and clinical longevity. Cerâmica. 2013. 59:633-639.

Bomicke, W.; Schurzb, A.; Krisam, J.; Rammelsbergd, P.; Ruese, S. Durability of Resin-Zirconia Bonds Produced Using Methods Available in Dental Practice. J Adhes Dent. 2016; 18:17-27.

Cvikl, B.; Dragicb, M.; Franzc, A.; Raabe, M.; Gruber, R.; Moritz, A. Long-term Storage Affects Adhesion Between Titanium and Zirconia Using Resin Cements. J Adhes Dent. 2014; 16: 459-464.

I According to the Standardization Manual for Dissertations and Theses of Faculdade Sao Leopoldo de Mandic of 2014, based on Vancouver style, and abbreviation of journal titles in accordance with Index Medicus.

Della Bona, A.; Pecho, O.E.; Alessandretti, R. Zirconia as a Dental Biomaterial. Materials. 2015; 8:4978-4991.

El-Ghany OSA, Sherief AH. Zirconia based ceramics, some clinical and biological aspects: Review. Future Dental Journal. 2016. 2: 55-64.

Fragoso, W.S.;Henriques, G.E.P.;Contreras, E.F.R.; Mesquita, M.F. The influence of mold temperature on the fit of cast crowns with commercially pure titanium. Braz Oral Res. 2005; 19(2):139-43.

Gomes AL, Oyagü RC, Lynch CD, Montero J,Albaladejo A. Influence of sandblasting granulometry and resin cement composition on microtensile bond strength to zirconia ceramic for dental prosthetic frameworks. Journal of Dentistry. 2013; 41: 31 - 41.

Guilardi LF, Pereira GKR, Gündel A, Rippe MP, Valandro LF. Surface micromorphology, phase transformation, and mechanical reliability of ground and aged monolithic zirconia ceramic. Journal of the mechanical behavior of biomedical materials. 2017. 65:849-856.

Hallmann L, Ulmer P, Lehmann F, Wile S, Polanski O, Johannes M, Kobe S, Totenberg T, Bornholdt S, Haase F, Kersten H, Kern M. Effect of surface modifications on the bond strengthof zirconia ceramic with resin cement Dental Materials. 2016. 32:631-639.

Inokoshi M, Munck JD, Minakuchi S, Meerbeek BV Meta-analysis of Bonding Effectiveness to Zirconia Ceramics. J Dent Res. 2014. 93 (4):329-334.

Kawai, N.; J.L.; Youmaru, H.Y.; Shinya, A.; Shinya, A. Effects of three luting agents and cyclic impact loading on shear bond strengths to zirconia with tribochemical treatment. Journal of Dental Sciences. 2012; 7: 118 - 124.

Kern M, Thompson VP. Effects of sandblasting and silica-coating procedures on pure titanium. J. Dent. 1994; 22: 300-306.

Kim MJ, Kim YK, Kim KH, Kwon TY. Shear bond strengths of various luting cements to zirconia ceramic: Surface chemical aspects. Journal of Dentistry. 2011; 39: 795 - 803.

Lung CYK, Liu D, Matinlinna JP. Surface treatment of titanium by a polydimethylsiloxane coating on bond strength of resin to titanium. Journal of the Mechanical behavior of biomedical materials. 2015. 41:168 - 176.

Lung CYK, Matinlinna JP. Aspects of silane coupling agents and surface conditioning in dentistry: An overview. Dental Materials. 2012;28: 467-477.

Luthardt, R.G.; Holzhüter, M.S.; Rudolph, H.; Herold, V.; Walter, M.H. CAD/CAM-machining effects on Y-TZP zirconia. Dental Materials. 2003; 20: 655-662.

Luthy, H; Loeffel, O; Hammerle C.H.F. Effect of thermocycling on bond strength of luting cements to zirconia ceramic. Dental Materials, 2006; 22:195-200.

Luthra R, Kaur P. An insight into current concepts and techniques in resin bonding to high strength ceramics. Australian Dental Journal. 2016. 61:163-173.

Manicone, P.F.;, Iommetti, R.P.;, R.;Raffaelli, L. An overview of zirconia ceramics: Basic properties and clinical applications. Journal of dentistry. 2007; 35:819 - 826.

Matinlinna JP, Heikkinen T, Ozcan M, Lassila LVJ, Vallittu PK. Evaluation of resin adhesion to zirconia ceramic using some organosilanes. Dental Materials. 2006; 22: 824-831. (a).

Matinlinna JP, Lassila LVJ, Vallittu PK. Evaluation of five dental silanes on bonding a luting cement onto silica-coated titanium. Journal of Dentistry. 2006; 34: 721 - 726. (b).

Matinlinna JP, Lassila LVJ, Vallittu PK. The effect of a novel silane blend system on resin bond strength to silica-coated Ti substrate. Journal of Dentistry. 2006; 34: 436 - 443. (c).

Mirmohammadi H, Aboushelib MN, Kleverlaan CJ, de Jager N, Feilzer AJ. The influence of rotating fatigue on the bond strength of zirconia-composite interfaces. Dent Mater. 2010 Jul; 26(7):627-33.

Miyazaki T, Nakamura T, Matsumura H, Ban S, Kobayashi T. Current status of zirconia restoration. Journal Prosthodontics Res. 2013; 57. 236 - 261.

Mosele JC, Borba M. Effect of particle sandblasting on the bond strength and mechanical behavior of zirconia-based ceramics - Review. Cerâmica. 2014. 60:179186.

Nettleship I, Stevens R. Tetragonal Zirconia Polycrystal (TZP) - A review". Int J High Technol Ceramics. 1987; 3:1-32.

Ozcan M, Vallittu PK. Effect of surface conditioning methods on the bond strength of luting cement to ceramics. Dental Materials. 2003 19: 725-731.

Ozcan M & Mira Bernasconi W. Adhesion to Zirconia Used for Dental Restorations: A Systematic Review and Meta-Analysis. Journal Adhes Dent. 2015. 17: 7-26.

Oyagüe, R.C.; Monticelli, F.; Toledano, M.; Estrella Osorio, E.; Ferrari, M.; Osorio, R. Influence of surface treatments and resin cement selection on bonding to densely-sintered zirconium-oxide ceramic. Dental Materials. 2009; 25: 172-179.

Papia E, Larsson C, du Toit M, Vult von Steyern P. 2014. Bonding between oxide ceramics and adhesive cement systems: A systematic review. Journal Biomed Mater

Research. 2014. 102B:395-413.

Piascik JR, Swift EJ, Thompson JY, Grego S, Stoner BR. Surface modification for enhanced silanation of zirconia ceramics. dental materials. 2009; 25:1116-1121.

Piconi C, Maccauro G. Zirconia as a ceramic biomaterial. Biomaterial. 1999; 20(1): 1- 25.

Pozzobon JL, Pereira GKR, Wandscher VF, Dorneles LS, Valandro LF. Mechanical behavior of Ytria-stabilized tetragonal zirconia polycrystalline ceramic after different zirconia surface treatments. Materials Science and Engineering. 2017. C 77:828835.

Qeblawi,D.M.; Munoz, C.A.; Brewer,J.D.; Jr, E.A.M. The effect of zirconia surface treatment on flexural strength and shear bond strength to a resin Cement. J Prosthet Dent. 2010. 103:210-220.

Shahin R, Kern M. Effect of air-abrasion on the retention of zirconia ceramic crowns luted with different cements before and after artificial aging. Dental Materials; 2010 26: 922-928.

Schneider R, Goes MF, Henriques GEP, Chan DCN. Tensile bond strength of dual curing resin-based cements to commercially pure titanium. dental materials. 2007; 23: 81-87.

Smith RL, Villanueva C, Rothrock JK, Garcia-Godoy CE, Stoner BR, Piascik JR, Thompson JY. Long-term microtensile bond strength of surface modified Zirconia. Dental materials. 2011; 27: 779-785.

Souza G, Hennig D, Aggarwal A, Tam LE. The use of MDP-based materials for bonding to zirconia. J Prosthet Dent. 2014. 112:895-902.

Satake A, Figueiredo JLG, Zaia WLS. Influence of surface treatments on the bond strength of zirconia ceramics. Revista Dental Press Estética. 2015, April-June. 12 (2):71-9.

Sundh A, Sjogren G. Fracture resistance of all-ceramic zirconia bridges with differing phase stabilizers and quality of sintering. Dent Mater. 2006 Aug; 22(8):778-84.

Taira Y, Matsumura H, Yoshida K, Tanaka T, Atsuta M. Influence of surface oxidation of titanium on Adhesion. Journal of Dentistry. 1998; 26 (1) 69-73.

Thompson JY, Brian R, Stoner BR, Piascik JR, Smith R. Adhesion/ Cementation to zirconia and other non- silicate ceramics: where are they now? Dent Mater. 2011; 27(1):71-82.

Tsuchimoto Y, Yoshida Y, Takeuchi M, Mine A, Yatani H, Tagawa Y. Effect of surface pre-treatment on durability of resin-based cements bonded to titanium. Dental Materials. 2006; 22: 545-552.

Tzanakakis EGC, Tzoutzas LG, Koidis PT. Is there a potential for durable adhesion to zirconia restorations? A systematic review. J Prosthet Dent. 2016. 115:9-19.

Wolfart, M; Lehmann, F.; Wolfart, S.; Kern, M. Durability of the resin bond strength to zirconia ceramic after using different surface conditioning methods. Dental Materials. 2007; 23: 45-50.

Yang, B.; Barloi, A.; Kern, M. Influence of air-abrasion on zirconia ceramic bonding using an adhesive composite resin. Dental Materials. 2010; 26: 44-50.

Yun JY, Ha SR, Lee JB, Kim SH. Effect of sandblasting and various metal primers on the shear bond strength of resin cement to Y-TZP ceramic. Dental Materials. 2010. 26: 650-658.

Zhao L, Jian YT, Wang XD, Zhao K. Bond strength of primer/cement systems to zirconia subjected to artificial aging. J Prosthet Dent. 2016. 116:790-796.

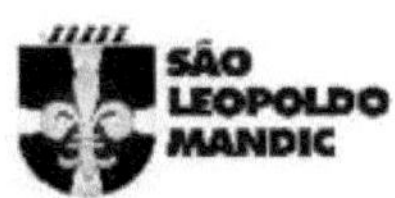

São Leopoldo Mandic

Centro de Pós-Graduação

Comunicado de Dispensa de Submissão ao Comitê

Campinas, 19 de dezembro de 2013.

Ao(a) RA

C.D. Rodrigo Giuberti 1117525

Curso: Prótese Dentária

Comitê:

Prezado(a) Aluno(a):

O projeto abaixo descrito, apresentado ao respectivo Comitê de Ética, nesta Instituição, foi dispensado de ser submetido à análise, por tratar-se exclusivamente de pesquisa laboratorial, sem envolvimento de seres humanos ou materiais.

Número do Protocolo: 2013/0159

Data entrada do Projeto: 01/12/2013

Data da Reunião do Comitê: 09/12/2013

Orientação por: Fabiano Perez

Projeto: *Resistência de união do cimento resinoso a superfície do titânio e zircônia tratado e não tratado*

Cordialmente,

Profa Dra Fernanda Lopes da Cunha
Presidente do Comitê de Ética em Pesquisa

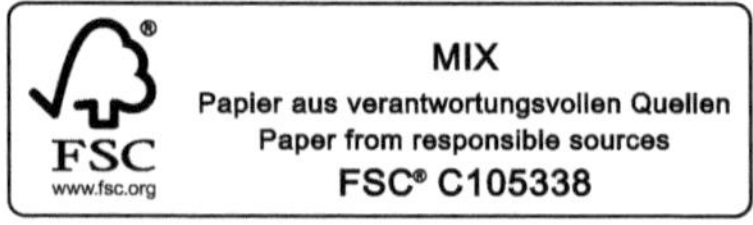

Printed by Books on Demand GmbH, Norderstedt / Germany